Medical Quotations

by Eminent Physicians and Philosophers

FOURTH EDITION

Medical Quotations

by Eminent Physicians and Philosophers

FOURTH EDITION

Meharban Singh
MD, FAMS, FIAP, FIMSA, FNNF, Hony. FAAP

Former Professor and Head
Department of Pediatrics and Neonatal Division
WHO Collaborating Center for Training and
Research in Newborn Care
All India Institute of Medical Sciences
New Delhi

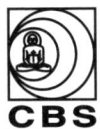

CBS

CBS Publishers & Distributors Pvt Ltd

New Delhi • Bengaluru • Chennai • Kochi • Kolkata • Mumbai
Hyderabad • Nagpur • Patna • Pune • Vijayawada

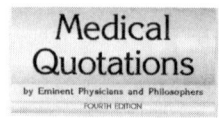

Medical Quotations
by Eminent Physicians and Philosophers
FOURTH EDITION

ISBN: 978-81-239-2882-1

Copyright © Meharban Singh

Fourth Edition: **2016**

First Edition: August 2003
Second Edition: October 2008
Third Edition: April 2013

Published by Satish Kumar Jain and Produced by Varun Jain for
CBS Publishers & Distributors Pvt Ltd
4819/XI Prahlad Street, 24 Ansari Road, Daryaganj, New Delhi 110 002, India.
Ph: 23289259, 23266861, 23266867   Website: www.cbspd.com
Fax: 011-23243014   e-mail: delhi@cbspd.com; cbspubs@airtelmail.in.
Corporate Office: 204 FIE, Industrial Area, Patparganj, Delhi 110 092
Ph: 4934 4934   Fax: 4934 4935   e-mail: publishing@cbspd.com; publicity@cbspd.com

Branches

- **Bengaluru:** Seema House 2975, 17th Cross, K.R. Road,
  Banasankari 2nd Stage, Bengaluru 560 070, Karnataka
  Ph: +91-80-26771678/79   Fax: +91-80-26771680   e-mail: bangalore@cbspd.com
- **Chennai:** No. 7, Subbaraya Street, Shenoy Nagar, Chennai 600 030,
  Tamil Nadu
  Ph: +91-44-26680620/26681266   Fax: +91-44-42032115   e-mail: chennai@cbspd.com
- **Kochi:** Ashana House, 39/1904, AM Thomas Road, Valanjambalam,
  Eranakulam 682 018, Kochi, Kerala
  Ph: +91-484-4059061-62-64-65   Fax: +91-484-4059065   e-mail: kochi@cbspd.com
- **Kolkata:** No. 6/B, Ground Floor, Rameswar Shaw Road, Kolkata-700014
  (West Bengal), India
  Ph: +91-33-2289-1126, 2289-1127, 2289-1128   e-mail: kolkata@cbspd.com
- **Mumbai:** 83-C, Dr E Moses Road, Worli, Mumbai-400018, Maharashtra
  Ph: +91-22-24902340/41   Fax: +91-22-24902342   e-mail: mumbai@cbspd.com

Representatives

- **Hyderabad**   0-9885175004
- **Pune**   0-9623451994
- **Nagpur**   0-9021734563
- **Vijayawada**   0-9000660880
- **Patna**   0-9334159340

Printed at Magic International Pvt. Ltd. Greater Noida, UP

to

*philosophers, polymaths
and medicalmen of eminence*

Preface to the Fourth Edition

The third edition of the book has been acclaimed as a unique "first of its kind" compendium of medical quotations and aphorisms by medical teachers, philosophers and men of wisdom. This has prompted and encouraged the Editor to bring out a revised, updated and an enlarged version. The earlier format of subjectwise classification of quotations has been maintained by incorporation of 175 additional sayings, proverbs, quotations, aphorisms, apothegms and statements by eminent medicalmen, thinkers, philosophers, scientists, clerics and politicians. The format, composing and quality of production have been improved to make it more reader-friendly. I am confident that the revised compendium of medical quotations would satisfy the felt needs of medical teachers and writers to have an easy access to a large number of sayings and aphorisms to inspire their orations and writings.

The cover design has been created by my granddaughter Ms Ishita Singh.

Meharban Singh

Child Care Center
625, Arun Vihar, Sector 37
Noida 201 301
Tel: 0120-4346451, 9818888772
e-mail: drmbsk@gmail.com

Preface to the First Edition

There are occasions when we wish to recall memorable phrases and quotations while writing a speech or giving a lecture. The lack of any standard publication on medical quotations in the Indian or international market, inspired me to collect, collate and create an handy manual of medical quotations by eminent physicians and philosophers. A brief chapter on Historical Milestones in Medicine gives a glimpse of Medical Eras and provides a brief life sketch and contributions of medicalmen of eminence. The quotations have been arranged subjectwise, under 26 subtitles for ease of retrieval to serve the needs of the readers.

The wisdom of the wise and experience of the sages are perpetuated by their quotations and sayings over the ages. The quotations provide a treasurehouse of penetrating wisdom, beautiful thought, a vision and at times an outstanding wit or humor of a sharp mind. A quotation in a speech, article or a book lends authority and aura to the speaker or writer and ignites the minds of listeners and readers.

I have gleaned through a large number of writings and teachings of the world's greatest minds, to extract a storehouse of their encapsulated wisdom expressed in the form of their famous aphorisms and quotations. The life is short and knowledge is like an ocean and it is impossible to explore and fathom its expanse and depth to the full. It is possible I may have missed some of the memorable quotations and sayings and I would like to request the readers to send me any other memorable medical quotations that they are aware of or their own catchy quotations for inclusion in the next edition of the book. I would like to take this opportunity to express my special appreciation to my friend Dr Doug McMillan for sending me some publications of Sir William Osler, the greatest medical writer of the millennium. I do hope that this compendium of medical quotations would fulfill your felt need to have a ready access to a treasurehouse of medical sayings and aphorisms that you can effectively harness to enliven your orations and writings.

Meharban Singh MD

Abbreviations Used for Gregorian or Christian Calendar

BC:	Before Christ
AD:	Anno Domino, i.e. in the year of the Lord
BCE:	Before the Common Era or Christian Era
CE:	Common Era or Christian Era
1st millennium:	1–1000 CE
2nd millennium:	1001–2000 CE
3rd millennium:	2001–3000 CE
Century:	100-year period
21st century:	Started on 1st January 2001

Note: BC and AD have been used to express calendar years in the book.

Contents

Historical Milestones in Medicine

1. *The Ancient Middle East* Herodotus and Diodorus Sicihas recorded historical medical events of Egyptians; Greeks and Romans during 1320 BC–1200 BC. The earliest Babylonian medical text, the Diagnostic Handbook was written by Esagil-kin-apli of Borsippa during the reign of king Adab-apla-iddina (1069 BC–1046 BC). The symptoms and diseases were treated with therapeutic means such as bandages, herbs and creams.

2. *Ancient Persian and Jewish Medicine* They had a common origin, which was recorded in the sacred persian book, The Avesta. In ancient times, medicine and religion were closely connected. The priests were the custodians of public health. Jews had high regard for physicians and considered them as the instrument through whom God could effect the cure. Jews had long line of rabbi-physicians and medicine was governed by Biblical and Talmudic laws. The prevailing superstitions and beliefs in magic medicine were far less accepted and practiced by Jews. Jewish physicians had special consideration for the poor and needy but free medical service was not approved because they believed that "a physician who takes nothing is worth nothing". The salient medical writings of this period included. Apocryphal books,

Graeco-Roman writings of Jews and non-Jews, the Misnah, the Jerusalem and Babylonian Talmuds, the Midrashim. Over the years, Jews have excelled in medical research and they have bagged over 20% of all Nobel Prizes.

The ancient Persian medicine dates back to Mesopotamian period (3000 BC) and it is as old and as rich as its civilization. The earliest practices of ancient Iranian medicine have been documented in The Avesta and other Zoroastrian religious texts. These books and texts laid great importance to personal hygiene, public health and prevention of contagious disorders. The best teachers of medicine and astrology in Iran were Magi and Mobeds. Avestan texts list a large number of herbs and plants with medicinal values.

3. **Ancient Indian Medicine** Ayurveda, a system of traditional medicine native to India, had its origin during the vedic period (1700 BC–1100 BC). In Sanskrit, the words *ayus* means longevity and *veda* means knowledge or science. Ayurveda believed in existence of "five elements", i.e. *Prithvi* (earth), *Jala* (water), *Agni* (fire), *Vayu* (air) and *Akasa* (sky) that compose the universe including the human body. Ayurveda attributed illness to an imbalance between three *doshas* or bioenergies, *vata* (ether or air), *pitta* (bile or fire and water) and *kapha* (phlegm or water and earth). Agnivesa wrote the earliest medical encyclopedia in 800 BC under the guidance of the ancient physician Atreya. Charaka revised and updated the treatise which came to be known as *Charaka Samhita*. Sushruta wrote a surgical compendium called *Sushruta Samhita*. The ancient Indians were centuries ahead of all other civilizations in the field of plastic surgery, performing operations to restore the shape of nose. Dhanvantri, the Hindu god of Ayurveda, is worshipped by its practitioners. During Indian Sultanate

and Moghul period, Unani medicine, another form of alternative medicine, became popular by virtue of royal patronage.

4. *Traditional Chinese Medicine* Chinese medicine is based on the principles of *yang* (positive or masculine) and *yin* (passive or feminine) energies. It was believed that illness was caused by imbalance of two forces while death occurred when they ceased to flow. The outstanding ancient Chinese medical books include *Pen Tsao Ching* or Herbal by Shen Nung and *Nei Ching* or Book of Medicine by Hwang Ti (2698 BC–2598 BC). Acupuncture was introduced with the idea of removing any obstruction in *chin* and *loh* or sun, the vessels carrying two vital principles, blood and air during T'ang Dynasty (618 AD–906 AD). An outstanding 52 volumes book called *Pen T'sao Kang Mu* or Great Herbal Medicine published in 1552 AD is a most comprehensive treatise on herbal medicine.

5. *Ancient Greek Medicine* Hellenic medicine for the first time became a science as well as an art. Many of the Greek gods came to be identified with healing—Apollo, Aremis, Athene, and Aphrodite. The first Greek medical school was opened in Cnidus in 700 BC. Alcmaeon worked at this school and published his monumental anatomical work. Hippocrates, Father of modern Medicine, established his own medical school at Cos. The Hippocratic oath, which is still taken by doctors on graduation, was written in Greek in the 5th century BC. During this period Galen was one of the greatest surgeons who performed complex surgeries on the brain and eyes. The writings of Greek physicians, Hippocrates, Galen and others had a lasting influence on Islamic medicine and medieval European medicine until many of their findings eventually became obsolete from the

14th century onwards. The mythological figure Asclepius (770 BC) is credited to have a large family and his sons were the gods of surgeons and physicians while his daughters called Panacea provided cure for everything and Hygieia looked after public health. Asclepius was represented by the sacred sign of god of healing in the form of a serpent coiled around a rod or staff.

6. *The Graeco-Italian School* Pythogoras (580 BC–489 BC) was the founder of Graeco-Italian school and introduced the concept of scientific medicine. It was postulated that ill health depended upon opposite elements like hot and cold, wet and dry, sweet and sour and so on. Empedocles of Agrigentum (500 BC–430 BC) believed that world is made up of four elements—earth, air, fire and water, and their balance is crucial for maintenance of health.

7. *Ancient Egyptian Medicine* Ancient Egypts mostly dealt with magic, witchcraft and supernatural remedies. They gradually developed practical knowledge in the fields of anatomy, public health and clinical diagnostics. Herodotus described the Egyptians as the "most healthiest of all men" by virtue of their notable public health system. Medical information compiled in the Edwin Smith Papyrus probably dates back to as early as 1600 BC. Imhotep in the 3rd Dynasty is credited to be the founder of ancient Egyptian medicine and original author of *Edwin Smith Papyrus*. Kahun Gynecological Papyrus dates back to 1800 BC and is believed to be the first text dealing with diseases of women and pregnancy disorders. Medical Institutes, referred to as Houses of Life were established in Egypt as early as the 1st Dynasty. The earliest known physician of ancient Egypt in 27th century BCE is believed to be Hesy-Ra, who was "Chief Dentist and Physician" to king Djoser. The earliest known woman physician Peseshet, practiced in Ancient Egypt at the time of 4th Dynasty.

8. *Middle ages or Medieval period (500 AD–1500 AD)* It began with the collapse of Western Roman Empire and merged with Renaissance and Age of Discovery (14th–17th century), which is a bridge between the middle ages and modern period. The surgical practices inherited from the ancient masters were improved and documented in Rogerius's the practice of surgery. The formal systematic training of physicians began around 1220 AD in Italy. During the Renaissance, the understanding of anatomy improved and the microscope was invented. The germ theory of disease in the 19th century lead to prevention and cures of many infectious diseases.

PHILOSOPHERS AND MEDICAL MEN OF EMINENCE

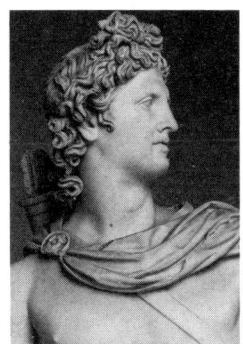

Apollo was the Greek god of sun, prophecy, poetry, music, archery and healing. He was the son of Zeus and Leto and had a twin sister Artemis. He was an attractive handsome athletic young man with curly golden hair. Apollo never married but had many lovers and mistresses and sired many sons including the famous god of healing Asclepius.

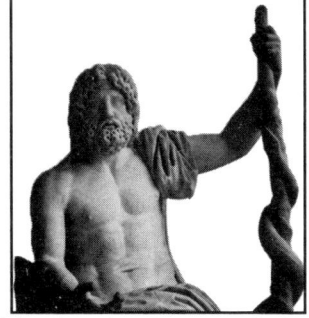

Asclepius is the Greek god of health and healing. He was the son of Apollo, the Greek sun god. His mother died when he was still in her womb. He cried aloud when his mother's body was placed on the funeral pyre. Apollo cut the womb and pulled out the unborn child and declared that this son of his, Asclepius, would be responsible for the human fight against disease and death. Apollo took the baby to Centaur Chiron who raised Asclepius and taught him the art of medicine.

Imhotep (2650 BC–2600 BC), an eminent Egyptian polymath is considered to be the first physician in ancient world. He was called *Imuthes* by Greeks. He was considered as eminent as Asclepius. There is compelling evidence that Joseph of Bible and Imhotep were the same person. He was chief architect, high priest, astrologer, scribe and 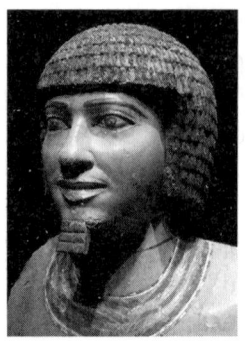 physician to king Pharaoh Djoser. He is the author of a medical treatise *Edwin Smith Papyrus* containing anatomical observations, ailments and cures. He has been given the status of a deity of medicine and healing. According to Sir William Osler, Imhotep was indeed the "Father of Medicine" who freed medicine from antiquity and witchcraft.

Hippocrates (460 BC–370 BC), the Father of modern Medicine was born on the Island of Kos or Cos, Greece and wrote *Corpus Hippocraticum* incorporating Hippocratic oath, 70 books and 406 sayings in the famous book of Aphorisms. He opposed age old Greek thoughts in medicine, for which he was 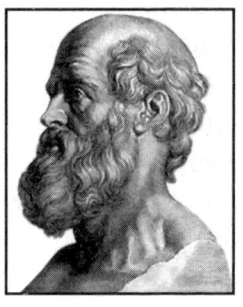 imprisoned for 20 years, where he wrote his famous medical works *"The Complicated Body"*. He separated the discipline of medicine from religion and was the first physician who believed that disease was not due to punishment inflicted by the gods but an outcome of faulty environmental factors, diet and living habits. He died at the outskirts of Larissa in 370 BC at the age of 90.

Sushruta or Susruta (around 600 BC), a contemporary of Charaka, is considered as Father of Plastic Surgery in India. The exact era of Sushruta is not known but it seems he preceded Charaka. He lived, taught and practiced his art on the bank of Ganges in the area that corresponds to present day city of Varanasi in North India. He was descendent of sage Vishvamitra. He learnt medicine and surgery at the feet of Divodasa Dhanvantri in his hermitage at Varanasi. He was most adept in 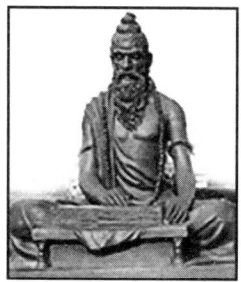 restructuring the cut or damaged nose. He is credited to be the first surgeon to undertake cesarean section, remove urinary stones, operate on cataract and set fractures. He used to give wine to his patients to numb the senses during the operation. He put forth the concept of asepsis several centuries before Joseph Lister. *Sushruta Samhita* gives a detailed description of 300 types of surgical operations and 120 types of surgical instruments, and classified human surgery into eight categories.

Charaka (Caraka) is known as the Father of Indian system of Medicine (Ayurveda) and lived most probably during 200 BC–300 BC. Nothing is known about the background of Acharya Charaka but it is believed that he was son of a sage who travelled from place to place (Charaka literally means "wandering" or "touring") on foot to 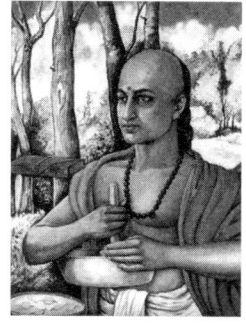 cure the suffering of the masses. He was the court physician of the Buddhist king Kanishka.

He was the first physician to present the concept of physiology, metabolism and immunity. According to him the body functions because it contains three *doshas* or humors, namely wind, bile and phlegm. These *doshas* are produced when *dhatus,* namely blood, flesh and marrow act upon the food eaten. The illness is caused when the balance among three *doshas* in a human body is disturbed. He knew the fundamentals of genetics and enumerated various factors which determine the sex of the child. He studied anatomy and embryology of the human body and mentioned that there are a total of 360 bones including teeth. He revised and updated the medical encylopedia written by Agnivesa in 800 BC, which came to be known as *Charaka Samhita*. It is an excellent Ayurvedic treatise in Sanskrit which was later translated into Persian, Arabic and Latin in 800 AD.

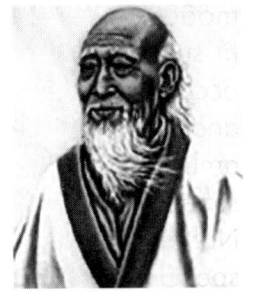

Lao Tzu (604 BC–531 BC), also known as LiErh or Laozi (old master), was born in the state of Ch'u in China. He is the Father of the Chinese spiritual tradition called Taoism. He was a contemporary of Confucius and wrote *Tao te Ching*, the main text highlighting the philosophy of Taoism.

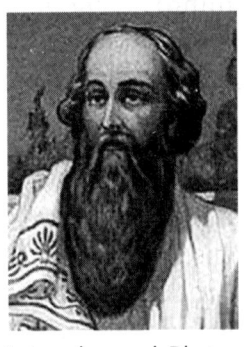

Pythogoras (570 BC–495 BC) was born in Samos, an island of Greece. He was a great mathematician, philosopher and religious teacher. He is remembered by his famous theorem in geometry, the "Pythagorean Theorem". His religious teachings centered on the doctrine of metapsychosis and believed in the doctrine of rebirth of person's soul. His ideas exercised a marked influence on Aristotle and Plato, and through them, all of western philosophy.

Gautama Buddha (563 BC–483 BC), also known as Siddhartha Gautama, Shakyamani, or simply Buddha (enlightened or awakened), was born on a full moon day at Lumbini, Nepal and grew up as a prince in Kapilavastu.

He was greatly touched and upset by human sufferings and left his palace at the age of 29 years to lead an ascetic life in search of perennial peace. He attained enlightenment or Nirvana at the age of 35 years, after meditating for 49 days under a pipal tree in Bodh Gaya, Bihar, India. He was a spiritual leader and founder of Buddhist religion.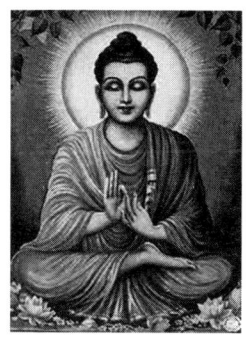

His teachings focus on the philosophy of a path of moderation or middle way, and four noble truths, i.e. (i) suffering is unavoidable part of existence, (ii) suffering occurs due to craving for sensuality, acquisition of identity and attempts for their annihilation, (iii) all desires and ambitions must be extinguished if you want freedom from suffering and (iv) suffering can be abolished by following Noble Eightfold Path of right view, right intention, right speech, right action, right livelihood, right effort, right mindfulness and right concentration. He achieved Parinirvana at Kushinagar, Uttar Pradesh, India after consuming his last meal offered by a disciple Cunda.

Confucius (551 BC–479 BC) was a great Chinese thinker, social philosopher and ethicist during Zhou dynasty. His influence on Chinese thought is considered as great as of Socrates in the west. He is called "The Greatest Master" by the Chinese people. His teachings were compiled in *The Analects* 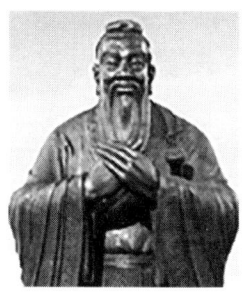 many years after his death. Confucius's family, the Kongs, has the longest recorded extant pedigree in the world spanning over 83 generations with 2 million registered descendants.

Socrates (470 BC–399 BC), a celebrated Greek philosopher was born at Athens in 470 BC. According to Cicero, "Socrates brought down philosophy from the heavens to the earth". A special Jury of the state issued an indictment against Socrates which stated, "Socrates is guilty of crime, first for not worshipping gods whom the city worships, and for 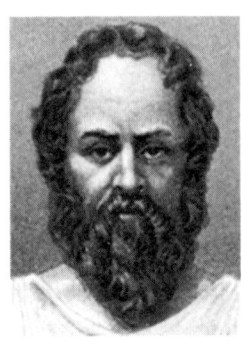 introducing new divinities of his own, next for corrupting the youth, the penalty due is death." He was executed by asking him to drink the poisonous extract of hemlock.

Plato (428 BC–348 BC) was a Greek philosopher and a mathematician. He was a student of Socrates and established an Academy in Athens. He is credited with a large number of philosophical dialogues. In his most influential work, The Republic, he extolled the virtues of justice, courage, 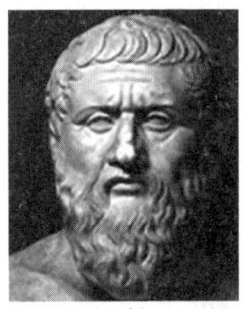 wisdom and moderation. He established a school of learning which was called Academy.

Aristotle (384 BC–322 BC) was a Greek philosopher and polymath, who was born in Stagira, small town in the northern coast of Greece. He was a pupil of Plato and tutor of Alexander the Great. He founded his own school, The Lyceum, in Athens where he spent most of his life studying, teaching and writing. He commented in his Rhetoric 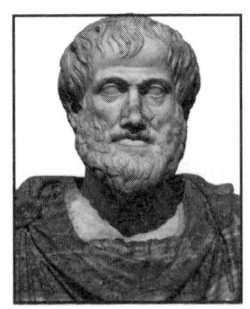 that a society cannot be happy unless its women are happy too.

Asclepiades (129 BC–40 BC) studied in Bithynia and was the first Greek doctor to succeed in Rome. He proposed a new theory of disease, based on the flow of atoms through pores in the body. He prescribed diet, exercise, walking, baths and massage instead of medicines. He believed doctors should act *"cito,* 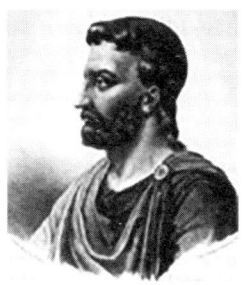 *tute et incunde"*—in a fast, safe and pleasant manner.

Marcus Tullius Cicero (106 BC–43 BC) was a Roman philosopher, statesman, lawyer and orator. He is widely considered as Rome's greatest orator and prose stylist. He popularised mnemonics as a memory booster. The English words Ciceronian (meaning 'eloquent') and Cicerone (meaning 'local guide') are derived from his name.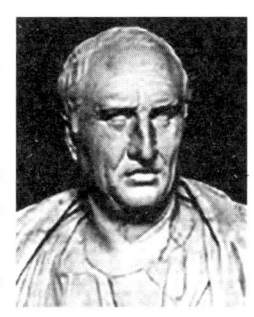

Aulus Cornelius Celsus (25 BC–45 AD) who lived at the start of Christian era, was the most famous of all Roman medical writers. His outstanding medical work, "De Medicine" was one of the best sources of medical knowledge during his time. Celsus described the four 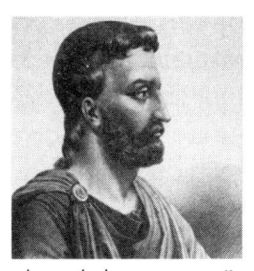 cardinal signs of inflammation—"rubor, color, dolor, tumor", i.e. redness, heat, pain and swelling.

Pedanius Discorides (40 AD–90 AD) was a Greek physician, pharmacologist and botanist. His five volume De Materia Medica described over 600 medicinal plants and was read for more than 1500 years. He is considered as the Father of modern Pharmacopoeia.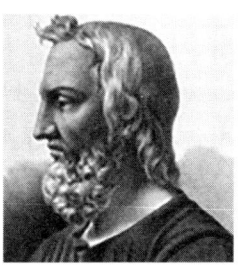

Soranus of Ephesus (98 AD–138 AD), a 2nd century Greek is considered as the Father of Obstetrics and Gynecology and wrote the four volume famous textbook entitled "Soranu's Gynecology" which remained popular for fifteen centuries. He wrote the biography of Hippocrates.

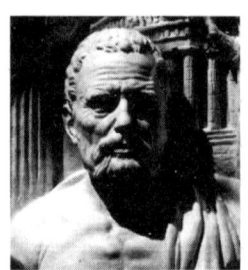

Claudius Galen (130 AD–203 AD) was born at Pergamon in Greece. Galen wrote over 400 publications, most of which were lost in a fire. He did some outstanding work on Anatomy and Physiology. He believed that venous and arterial systems were sealed and independent of each other.

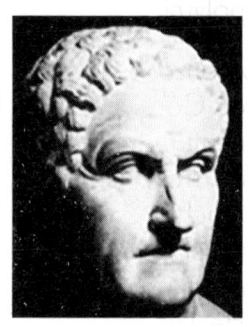

Rhazes or Razes (854 AD–925 AD) born as Abu Baker Muhammad Ibn Zakariya al-Razi, was a Persian from Tehran who studied medicine in Baghdad. He was a multifaceted personality (polymath) with interests in mathematics, astronomy, religion and philosophy; but over half of his 237 works dealt with medicine. He made numerous clinical observa-

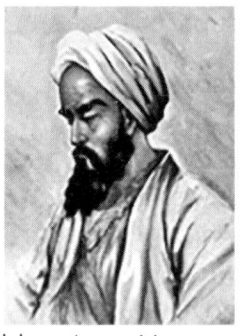

tions as a physician during Islamic Golden Age. He was the first physician to differentiate smallpox from measles. He is often called Father of Pediatrics for writing The Diseases of Children, the first book to deal with pediatrics as an independent field of medicine.

Avicenna or Ibu Ali Sina or Ibn Sina (980 AD–1037 AD) was born at Kharmaithen near Bukhara, Hamadan, Iran and became the most renowned Arab medical practitioner. He was a precocious child who could recite Quran at the age of 10 years. His most famous works are The Book of Healing and the five-volume al-Quanun (The Canon of Medicine) which served as a medical bible in the medical schools of the western world for several decades. He is regarded as the most famous and influential polymath of the Islamic Golden Age.

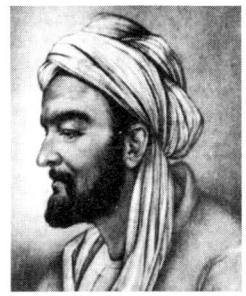

Avenzoar or Ibn Zuhr (1090 AD–1162 AD) of Cordoba was born in the twelfth century in Seville, Spain. He was non-conformist and challenged the teachings of Avicenna and Galen. His most celebrated pupil was Musa Ibn Maimun better known as Maimonides. He was a crusader against quackery and superstitious remedies.

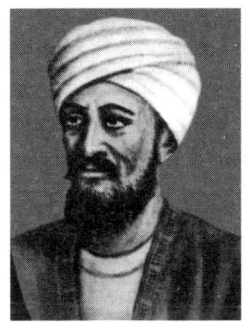

Moses ben Maimonides (1135 AD–1204 AD) also known as Musa Ibn Maymun or Moses ben Maimon was a Jewish philosopher, rabbi and physician who worked in Morocco and Egypt. He wrote ten medical texts in Arabic that have been translated into English by Jewish ethicist Fred Rosner.

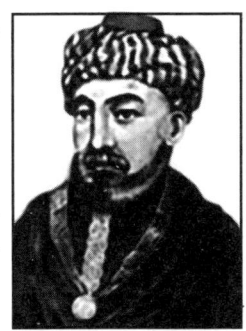

Mondino de Liuzzi (1270 AD–1326 AD) was an Italian physician who started systematic dissection at the university of Bologna and wrote a valuable textbook called Anathomia Corporis Humani. He was the first to introduce systematic study of anatomy and human dissection in the

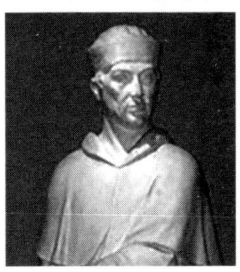

medical curriculum. He was regarded as a "divine master" and his observations recorded in Anathomia were considered as gospel truth.

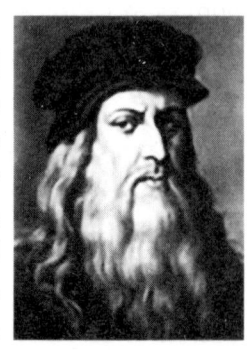

Leonardo da Vinci (1452 AD–1519 AD) was born to unmarried parents on April 15, 1452 near Vinci, Italy. He was recognised as a genius for his paintings (especially the Mona Lisa and The Last Supper) and drawings and also as an architect, engineer, scientist and inventor. He is considered by some the Father of Anatomy by virtue of his keen powers of observation and stupendous technical skills.

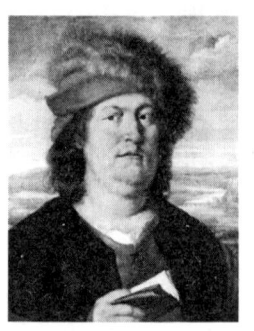

Paracelsus (1493 AD–1541 AD) was born in Einsiedeln in Switzerland and was a German-Swiss Renaissance physician, botanist, astrologer and occultist. He authored more than 300 works ranging from medicine to alchemy and metaphysics. He pioneered the use of chemicals and minerals in medicine. He discovered zinc which was initially named zink. He is often called the Father of Toxicology.

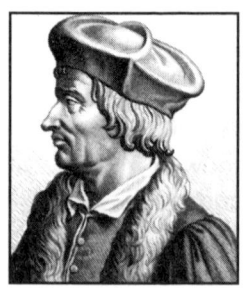

Jean Francois Fernel (1497 AD–1558 AD) was the greatest contemporary of Paracelsus who became professor of medicine in Paris and wrote a historical textbook *Universa Medica* which remained a standard text for the next two centuries. He introduced the term "physiology" to describe the study of body's functions. He was the first person to describe spinal canal. The lunar crater Fernelius is named after him.

Andreas Vesalius (1514 AD – 1564 AD) was 16th century Belgian physician who wrote seven books on the structure of human body called *De Humani Corporis Fabrica Libri Septem* which was printed in Basle. He laid the foundation of modern medicine and is truly the Father of Anatomy.

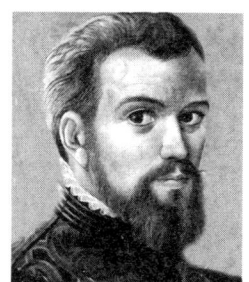

Ambroise Pare (1517 AD–1590 AD), a French national, is regarded as the founder of modern surgery and obstetrics and wrote an outstanding book *De la Generation de l'Homme*. He was a pioneer in the field of battle-field injuries and modern forensic pathology. He made outstanding contributions to create limb and ocular prostheses for victims of war.

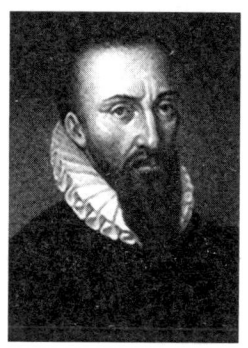

Galileo Galilei (1564 AD–1642 AD) was an Italian physicist, astronomer and philosopher who looked for an exact mathematical law governing every phenomenon and used research and science for measurement. He is considered as the Father of modern Science.

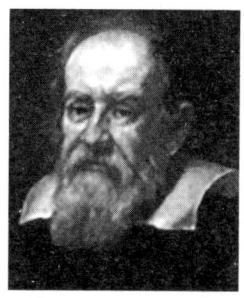

William Harvey (1578 AD–1657 AD) was an English physician who discovered the circulation of blood in 1616. He showed that flow of blood is continuous and always in one direction and the blood changed from the venous to the arterial in the lungs. He published his famous treatise on the motion of the heart and blood titled "De Motu Cordis" in 1628.

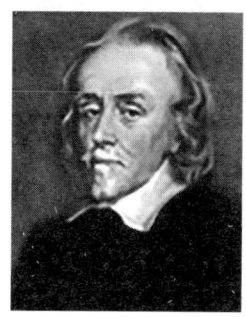

Thomas Sydenham (1624 AD – 1689 AD) was born on September 10, 1624 at Wynford Eagle in Dorset and was popularly called the "English Hippocrates". He shared the faith of Hippocrates in the healing powers of nature. Among his achievements was the discovery of a disease Sydenham chorea, also known as St. Vitus Dance.

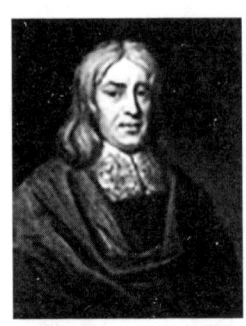

Robert Boyle (1627 AD–1691 AD) was an Anglo-Irish philosopher, chemist, physicist and inventor. He demonstrated that air was necessary for life as well as combustion, and that neither a flame nor an animal could survive in a vacuum. He is best known for Boyle's law which describes inversely proportional relationship between the absolute pressure and volume of a gas.

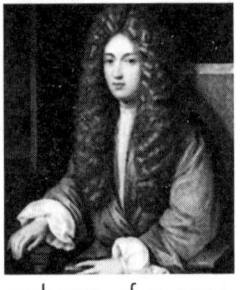

Marcello Malpighi (1628 AD–1694 AD) of Bologna, Italy is considered as the founder of microscopic anatomy of living tissues. His work on the capillaries complemented the discovery of circulation of the blood. Several microscopic anatomical structures are named after him including Malpighi layer in skin, two different Malpighian corpuscles in the kidneys and spleen.

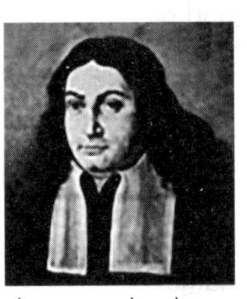

Giovanni Battista Morgagni (1682 AD– 1771 AD), professor of anatomy at university of Padua in Bologna, Italy is regarded as the founder of pathological anatomy. He published an outstanding book on the subject *De Sedibus et causis Morleorum* which gave a detailed account of sites and causes of diseases.

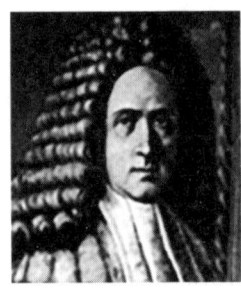

Herman Boerhaave (1688 AD–1738 AD), a Dutchman, was the greatest physician of the century who emphasized the importance of bedside teaching. He published *Institutiones Medicare*, a physiology textbook and *Aphorisms* which went through a large number of editions and translations.

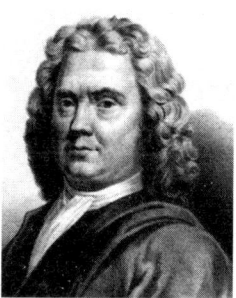

Francois-Marie Arouet or Voltaire (1694 AD–1778 AD) was born on November 21, 1694 in Paris, France. He was a renowned philosopher, literary genius and one of the greatest names of the French Enlightenment. He is credited with outstanding writings on history, culture, religion and philosophy under the pen name of Voltaire. He was known for his wit, poetry and playwrights. He was a rebel and one of the forerunners of French Revolution.

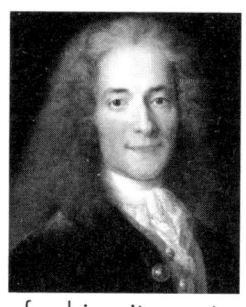

Carl von Linne or Linnaeus (1707 AD–1778 AD), a Swedish doctor and botanist, devised a system of classification of plants and animals and placed man in the order of primates with the name of *Homo Sapiens*. He is considered as Father of Taxonomy and Ecology.

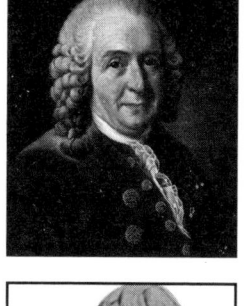

Franz Anton Mesmer (1734 AD–1815 AD) was born in Lake Boden in Germany. He went to Vienna to study theology, philosophy and law. He qualified medicine in Vienna and popularized magnetic therapy and mesmerism or hypnosis, i.e. healing by the power of imagination and trance.

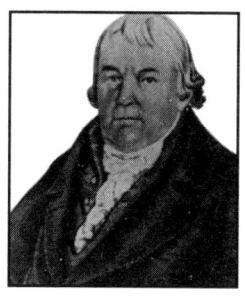

Edward Jenner (1749 AD–1823 AD) was an English physician who made an interesting observation that milkmaids who caught the cowpox virus did not suffer from smallpox. He launched a new era of preventive medicine by pioneering the use of cowpox vaccine to produce immunity against smallpox. 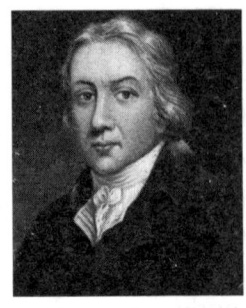 The dreaded disease was finally eradicated from the globe in 1979 by the universal immunization program.

Christian Friedrich Samuel Hahnemann (1755 AD–1843 AD), a German physician was born at Meissen, Saxony. He is the Father of Homeopathy and upheld the principle *"Similia Similibus Curantur"* (like is cured by like) after 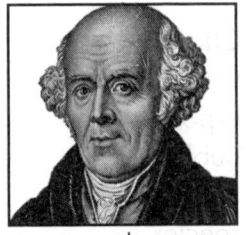 having experimented on himself with various medicines.

Humphry Davy (1778 AD–1829 AD) recognized the analgesic properties of nitrous oxide in 1799 and coined the term "laughing gas". He was an outstanding English chemist who discovered several alkalis and alkaline earth metals, and identified the elemental nature of chlorine and iodine.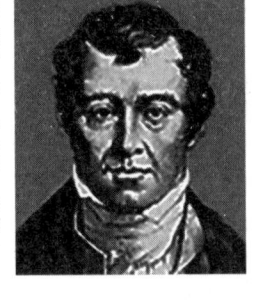

Rene-Theophile-Hyacinthe Laennec (1781 AD–1826 AD), a French physician is known as Father of Pulmonary Medicine. He popularized percussion and invented stethoscope for auscultation which has become a symbol of modern physicians. He coined the name cirrhosis for alcoholic damage to the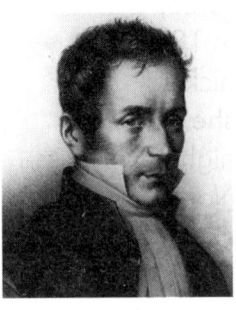

liver which is known as Laennec's cirrhosis. He served as a personal physician to Napolean Bonaparte.

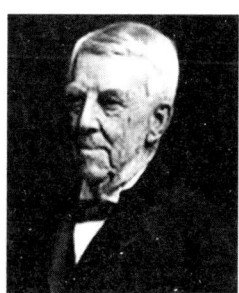

Oliver Wendell Holmes (1804 AD–1894 AD), an American clinician, poet and philosopher is credited for the discovery of anesthesia in 1840's. He is one of the best writers of 19th century and made outstanding contributions in the understanding of puerperal fever.

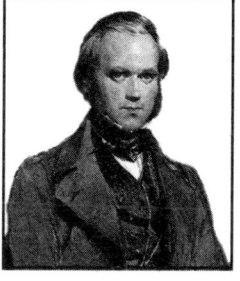

Charles Darwin (1809 AD–1882 AD), the great English naturalist and geologist, expounded the theory of evolution by publishing his work "On the Origin of Species". He propounded that all species of life have descended over a period of time from common ancestors by a process of natural selection.

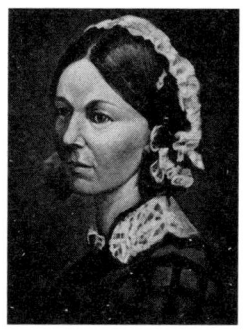

Florence Nightingale (1820 AD–1910 AD) was born to English parents in Florence, Italy on May 12, 1820. She made outstanding contributions as a nurse during the Crimean war between Russia and Turkey (supported by Britain and France) in 1853. During the war she gained the nickname, "The Lady with a Lamp" as she visited all the injured soldiers at night. She wrote two popular books, *Notes on Nursing and Notes on Hospitals*. She extolled the healing virtues of nature like fresh air, sunlight, plentiful space, nutritious food, warmth, clean surroundings and solitude. The Nightingale

Pledge taken by newly qualified nurses was named in her honor and the annual International Nurses Day is celebrated throughout the world on her birthday.

Rudolph Virchow (1821 AD–1902 AD), a German doctor, was the greatest nineteenth century pathologist who stated that diseases manifested in the cells and not in invisible and intangible humors. He is considered as the Father of modern Pathology and one of the founders of social medicine.

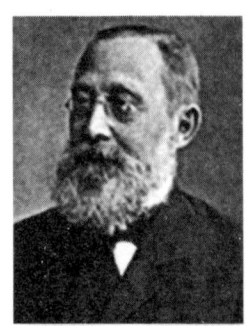

Gregor Mendel (1822 AD–1884 AD), an Austrian monk turned botanist, propounded the fundamental laws of genetics and Mendelian principles of inheritance of genetic disorders. His observations on pea plants in the monastery's garden became the foundation of modern genetics and the study of heredity and he is widely considered a pioneer in the field of genetics. He is known as Father of modern Genetics.

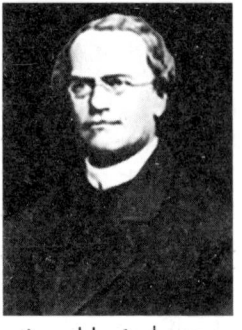

Louis Pasteur (1822 AD–1895 AD) was born on December 27, 1822 at Dole, France. He is considered as the Father of modern Microbiology. In his inaugural lecture at the university of Lille he made his famous remark: "In the field of observation, events favor only those who are prepared". He is a pioneer in the field of sterilization and pasteurization (making milk and wines safe for consumption) and created the first vaccine against rabies and anthrax.

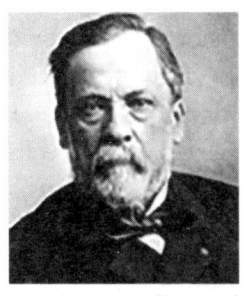

Joseph Lister (1827 AD–1912 AD) was a British surgeon who introduced the concept of disinfection of the surgical instruments with carbolic acid (phenol) at Glasgow and gave a boost to the safety of surgical procedures. He invented a pump to spray carbolic acid in the operation theaters. His principles 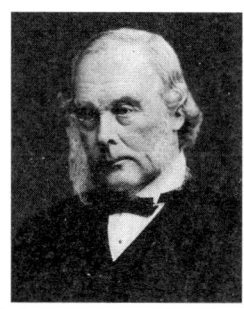 of antisepsis during surgery were widely accepted. The "Listerine" mouthwash is named after him.

Alfred Bernhard Nobel (1833 AD–1896 AD) was born on October 21, 1833 in Stockholm, Sweden. He was a multi-faceted personality, an outstanding business leader, engineer, chemist, scientist and inventor. He invented dynamite and other explosives and accumulated enormous fortune from 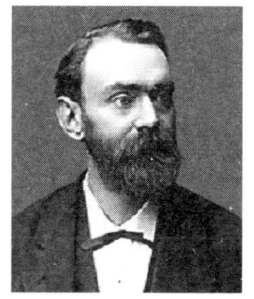 350 patents. In 1988, a French newspaper erroneously published his obituary (instead of his brother Ludvig who died), and condemned Alfred as "the merchant of death" for his invention of dynamite. He was greatly upset and did not want to be remembered as a dynamite inventor. He set aside bulk of his estate (equivalent of about US $ 472 million in 2012) to institute Nobel Prize awards for greatest achievements in various scientific fields throughout the world.

Robert Koch (1843 AD – 1910 AD) was a German physician who discovered *Mycobacterium tuberculosis, Cholera vibrio;* and *B. anthracis;* the etiological agents for tuberculosis, cholera and anthrax. He enunciated his own criteria (Koch's postulate) for suspecting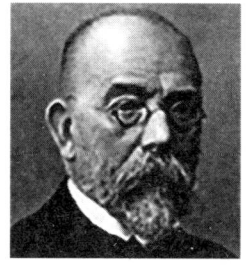

infectious etiology of a disease. He was awarded Nobel Prize in medicine or physiology in 1905 for his work on tuberculosis.

Wilhelm Konrad Roentgen (1845 AD–1923 AD), a German physicist, while conducting experiments involving the passage of electricity through vacuum tubes made a momentous chance discovery of X-rays in 1895. He received the Nobel Prize for physics in 1901.

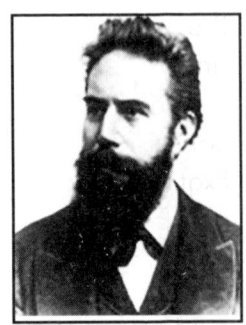

William Osler (1849 AD–1919 AD) was born at Bond Head, Ontario, Canada to English parents. He was the first Chairman of the Department of Medicine at Johns Hopkins University (1889–1905) and was subsequently invited to serve as Regius Professor of Medicine at Oxford. Osler Published his landmark textbook *The Principles and Practice of Medicine* in 1892, a lucid and literate work, that had enormous influence on medicine for over forty years.

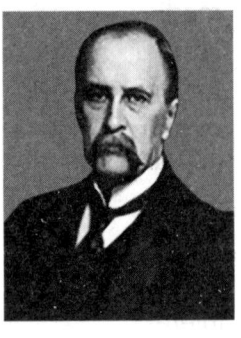

Paul Ehrlich (1854 AD–1915 AD), a German doctor, was an outstanding scientific genius who propounded the scientific basis for immunology and founded antimicrobial therapy. He received Nobel Prize for physiology or medicine for his discovery of effective treatment for syphilis.

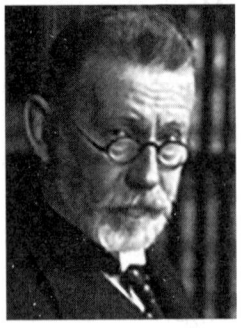

Sigmund Freud (1856 AD–939 AD), an Austrian neurologist postulated that many mental conditions have their roots in the life experiences and problems of the patient. He introduced psycho-analysis to unfold and bring out the unconscious beliefs into the realm of consciousness. He described gender 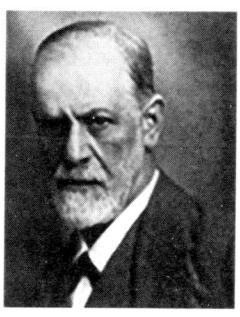 fixation of children with their parents as Oedipus complex and Electra complex.

Ronald Ross (1857 AD–1932 AD) was an Indian born (b. Almora) British medical doctor who received the Nobel Prize for physiology or medicine in 1902 for his work on malaria. His discovery of various stages of the malarial parasite in the gastrointestinal tract of mosquito laid the foundation for control of malaria. He worked in Indian Medical 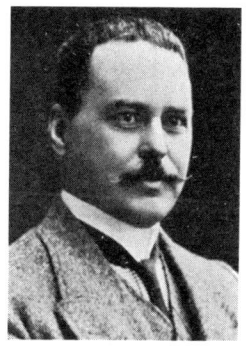 Service for 25 years. He was a polymath with wide ranging interests as an artist, mathematician and a writer of poems, novels and songs.

Marie Curie nee Maria Sklodowska (1867 AD–1934 AD) was born in Warsaw, Poland on November 7, 1867. She discovered radium and was awarded Nobel Prize in physics in 1903 and again in 1911 in chemistry for recognition of her work on radioactivity. She was the first woman to win a Nobel 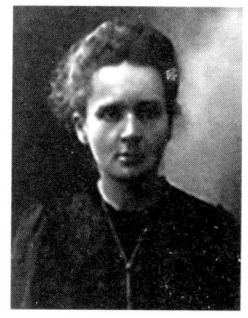 Prize and the only person to win the award in two different fields.

Harvey Williams Cushing (1869 AD– 1939 AD) was born on April 8, 1869 at Cleveland, Ohio. He is considered as the Father of modern Neurosurgery. He discovered the deadly Cushing disease. The Harvey Cushing Society, the first-of-its-kind neurosurgical association was established in his honor.

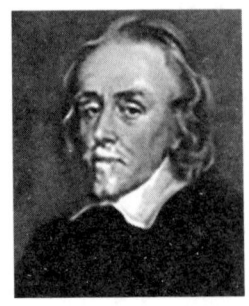

Ironically, he succumbed to a brain disorder, a cyst in the third ventricle.

Carl Jung (1875 AD–1961 AD) was a Swiss physician. He is the founder of analytical psychology and is often called "Darwin of the mind". He believed that everyone carries the repressed experiences and unpleasant memories in subconscious mind which are expressed through our behavior and dreams. He popularized psychoanalysis

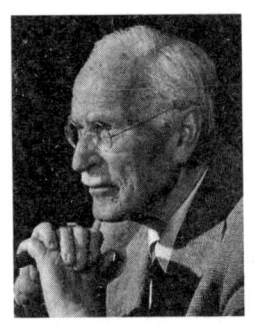

and analysis of dreams to cure people with disorders of mind.

Albert Einstein (1879 AD–1955 AD) was born to Jewish parents on March 14, 1879 at Ulm, Württemberg, Germany. He is considered as the most influential physicist of the 20th century who propounded the theory of relativity. He was awarded Nobel Prize for physics for his understanding of the photoelectric effect. Due to Nazi threat, he moved to

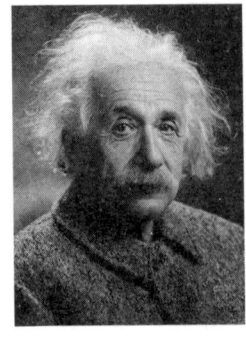

United States and became an American citizen in 1940.

Sir Alexander Fleming (1881 AD–1955 AD) was a Scottish biologist and pharmacologist. He discovered penicillin in 1928, which got nicknamed as "the wonder drug" and Fleming (along with Howard Florey and Ernst Boris Chain) was awarded Nobel Prize in medicine or physiology in 1945.

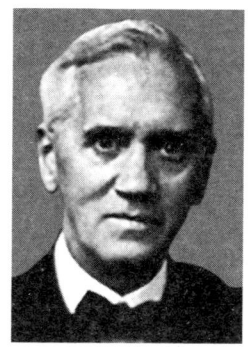

Frederick Grant Banting (1891 AD–1941 AD). He was born on November 14, 1891 in Alliston in Ontario. He had wide ranging interests and is best known for his discovery of wonder drug insulin. He is the youngest recipient of Nobel Prize in medicine or physiology at the age of 32 years. His name was etched into the Canadian Hall of Fame and a crater in the moon has been designated "Banting".

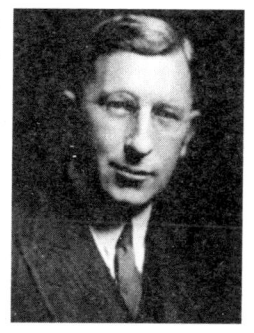

Ernst Ruska (1906 AD–1988 AD) was a German physicist who made the first electron microscope in 1930s to study subcellular biology. He demonstrated that a magnetic coil could act as an electron lens, and used several coils in a series to create the electron microscope. He was awarded Nobel Prize in physics in 1986, for his achievements in electron optics.

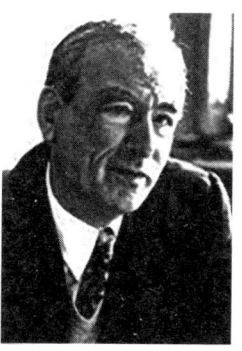

Christiaan Neethling Barnard (1922 AD–2001 AD) was a South African cardiac surgeon who performed the world's first successful human-to-human heart transplant, on 3rd December, 1967. The operation lasted for nine hours and was conducted by a team of 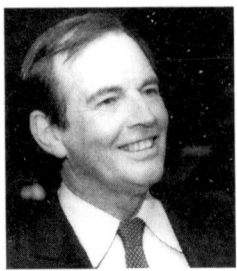 thirty people. He wrote several books including two autobiographies.

1

Art of Medicine

"From inability to let well alone, from too much zeal for the new and contempt for what is old, from putting knowledge before wisdom, science before art and cleverness before commonsense, treating patients as cases, from making the cure of the disease more grievous than endurance of the same, good Lord deliver us."

–Robert Hutchison

"......Our power to heal people and their lives seem to have diminished as dramatically as our power to cure diseases has increased. In the maze of scientific advances we have lost the human dimension."

–Bernie Siegel

"Good medicine is more than mere advanced knowledge, skills and drugs. It is an art to open the floodgates of psychic energy to catalyze the process of self healing. Awaken the powers of the patients to heal themselves. Energize the psycho-immuno-neurology axis by establishing communication with the inner self."

–Author Unknown

"Because all the sick do not recover, therefore, medicine is not an art."

–Cicero

"The physician must be compassionate, and must exhibit deep interest in the art and service of healing. Treatment of diseases consists in eliminating the factors underlying its causation, prescribing medicines or doing a surgical procedure, providing suitable diet, activity and regimen which will restore the balanced state of the body. It requires the combined efforts and synergy between the physician, nurse, patient and medicine."

–Charak Samhita

"The doctor who can no longer find time in his day for prayer and the inner life, time to prepare for his consultations in the presence of God and to seek His will for his patients, cannot bring to them the spiritual climate that is necessary if they are to open their hearts to him. Driven on by his devotion to the needs of his practice, he leads a fatiguing and unsatisfying life in which only more and more rarely does he find those peaceful moments in intimacy when he can provide what the patient most expects of him."

–Paul Tournier

"Life is short, art is long, opportunity is fleeting, experience is treacherous and judgement is difficult."

–Hippocrates

"The art of medicine cannot be inherited, nor can it be copied from books…"

–Paracelsus

"Nature, time and patience are the three great physicians."

–HG Bohn

"A physician who fails to enter the body of a patient with lamp of knowledge and understanding can never treat diseases. He should first study all the factors including environment, which influence a patients' disease, and then prescribe treatment. It is more important to prevent the occurrence of disease than to seek a cure."

–Charaka

"Wherever the art of medicine is loved, there is also a love of humanity."

–Hippocrates

"The physician must be able to tell the antecedents, know the present, foretell the future; must meditate on these things; and have two special objects in view with regard to diseases, namely to do well and to do no harm. The art consists in three things; the disease, the patient and the physician. The physician is the servant of the art and the patient must combat the disease along with the physician."

–Hippocrates

"Medicine is of all the arts the most noble, but owing to the ignorance of those who, inconsiderately, form a judgement of them, it is at present far behind all the other arts. Their mistake appears to me to arise principally from this, that in the cities there is no punishment connected with the practice of medicine except disgrace and that does not hurt those who are familiar with it...Physicians are many in title but very few in reality."

–Hippocrates

"...What happens then is like what happens when we separate a jigsaw puzzle into its five hundred pieces. The over-all picture disappears. This is the state of modern medicine. It has lost the sense of the unity of man. Such is the price it has paid for its scientific progress. It has sacrificed art to science."

–Paul Tournier

"Oh God, let my mind be ever clear and enlightened. By the bedside of patient, let no alien thought deflect it. Let everything that experience and scholarship have taught it be present in it and hinder it not in its tranquil work. For great and noble are those scientific judgements that serve the purpose of preserving health and lives of thy creatures..."

–Moimonides bin Musa

"Medicine is a science of uncertainty and art of probability."

–William Osler

"We profess to teach the principles and practice of medicine, or in other words, the science and art of medicine. Science is knowledge reduced to principles, art is knowledge reduced to practice. Your knowledge is useless unless you cultivate the art of healing. Unfortunately, the scientific man very often has the least amount of art, and he is totally unsuccessful in practice; and on the other hand, there may be much art based on an infinitesimal amount of knowledge, and yet it is sufficient to make its cultivator eminent."

–Samuel Wilks

"Irrespective of whatever cognitive quantum leaps may be made in the future, the physician of the 21st century shall continue to orchestrate with the melody of molecules, remain avidly attached to the music of mathematics, and shall get increasingly involved with the cosmology of computers. While doing so, his inherent capacity to develop an inner vision and in-depth perception, must go beyond the hitherto known frontiers of biosciences. Indeed this is where the sublime art of medicine surpasses the narrow confines of the biofrontiers of the science of medicine. This is also when a physician attains the divine gift of healing. Yet, how many strive for both? And how few achieve either!"

–JS Bajaj

"Medicine deals with states of health and disease in the human body. It is truism of philosophy that a complete knowledge of a thing can only be obtained by elucidating its causes and antecedents, provided, of course, such causes exist. In medicine, it is, therefore, necessary that causes of both health and disease should be determined."

—Avicenna

"The world does not need a new medicine. It needs doctors who know how to pray and obey God in their own lives. In such hands, medicine with all its modern resources, will bring forth fruits in abundance."

—Paul Tournier

"A good physician treats the disease, the great physician treats the patient who has the disease."

—William Osler

"Medical school teaches everything we need to know about writing prescriptions but nothing about understanding people. We need to show 'rational concern' and not 'detached concern' towards our patients."

—Franz Kafka

"Avoid intimacies with your patients, and visit them only in sickness."

—Benjamin Rush

"The art of medicine is valuable to us because it is conducive to health, not because of its scientific interest."

—Cicero

"For the art of medicine would not have been invented at first, nor would it have been made a subject of investigation (for there would have been no need of it) if when men are indisposed, the same food and other articles of regimen which they eat and drink when in good health were proper for them, and if no others were preferable to these. But now necessity itself made medicine to be sought out and discovered by men."

–Hippocrates

"The technical and diagnostic skills of a physician are no substitute for his bedside manners."

–Meharban Singh

"The aim of medicine is to prevent disease and prolong life, the ideal of medicine is to eliminate the need of a physician."

–William James Mayo

"The doctors most learned in theory are seldom the most skilled practitioners."

–Edme Pierre Beauchene

"To array a man's will against his sickness is the supreme art of medicine."

–Henry Ward Beecher

"An inquiring, analytical mind, an unquenchable thirst for new knowledge, and a heartfelt compassion for the ailing – these are prominent traits among the committed clinicians who have preserved the passion for medicine.

–Lois DeBakey

"The art of medicine consists in amusing the patient while nature cures the disease."

–Voltaire

"Medicine is not only a science; it is also an art. It does not consist of compounding pills and plasters; it deals with the very processes of life, which must be understood before they may be guided."

–Paracelsus

"Never forget that it is not a pneumonia, but a pneumonic man who is your patient."

—William Withey Gull

"The greatest mistake in the treatment of diseases is that there are physicians for the body and physicians for the soul, and the two cannot be separated."

—Plato

"While medicine is to be your vocation or calling, so to it that you have also an avocation—some intellectual pastime which may serve to keep you in touch with the world of art, of science or of letters."

—William Osler

"...In the physician or surgeon no quality takes rank with 'Imperturbability'."

—William Osler

"Oh the powers of nature. She knows what we need, but the doctors know nothing."

—Benvenuto Cellini

"....Thou shalt behave and act without arrogance and with undistracted mind, humility and constant reflection, thou shalt pray for the welfare of all creatures (not only your patients)......"

—Charaka

"Imperturbability... It is the quality which is most appreciated by the laity though often misunderstood by them; and the physician who has the misfortune to be without it, who betrays indecision and worry, and who shows that he is flustered and flurried in ordinary emergencies, loses rapidly the confidence of his patients."

—William Osler

"Over the years, the art to science ratio of medicine, has undergone a dramatic change. The medical pendulum has swung from the art to the science side. However, the best clinician is one, who is armed with the scientific knowledge, using excellent clinical judgement and practices with due compassion and understanding."

–NH Tucker

"For the most part, Western medicine doctors are not healers, preventers, listeners or educators. But they're damn good at saving life and other aspects kick the beam. It's about time we brought some balance back to the scale."

–Clair Todae

"We have to ask ourselves whether medicine is to remain a humanitarian and respected profession or a depersonalized science in the service of prolonging life rather than diminishing human suffering."

–Elisabeth Kübler-Ross

"The physicians of one class see the patients and go away merely prescribing the medicine. As they leave the room, they simply ask the patient to take the medicine. They are the poorest class of physicians."

–Ramakrishna

2

Brain–The Supreme Organ

"Your brain is far superior to the most advanced computer system in the world. A computer that came even close to matching an average human brain, would have to be at least the size of England."

–James Watson

"Our inner consciousness is an infallible guide to us and has infinite wisdom. Call it what you may—inner self, innate intelligence, superconscious, the source, your higher self— it doesn't matter. We call it your "intuition" or "inner-tuition" that keeps you focussed or "tuned-in.""

–Rex Johnson and David Swindley

"Our brains consist of two hemispheres. The left brain is responsible for logical and rational thinking while right brain governs the intuitive and creative faculties. The left brain communicates through use of numbers and language, the right by means of dreams, symbols and sudden flashes of insight."

–Roger Sperry

"Your brain is particularly vulnerable to oxygen free radical damage for two reasons. First, it is a hot bed of activity, it never stops working. Brain cells need a constant flow of blood and oxygen to produce energy, which increases the production of free radicals. Second, the brain is composed of 50 percent fat, which makes it vulnerable to lipid peroxidation."

–Lester Packer

"Research studies have conclusively shown that adding vitamins and minerals to the diets of children who have no obvious physical signs of nutrient deficiency can nevertheless produce an increase in their IQ scores."

–John Yudkin

"Aging of nervous system appears to involve a life-time of insults, many of which center around a common process; free radical generation and injury."

–Russel L. Blaylock

"The human brain starts working the moment you are born and never stops until you stand up to speak in public."

–George Jessel

"Human brain contains about 28 billion neurons. The neurons are interconnected through an amazing network of 100,000 miles of nerve fibers. It can process up to 30 billion bits of information per second with the 6,000 units of wiring and cabling. The information received by a neuron can spread to thousands of other neurons in a span of less than 20 milliseconds."

–Anthony Robbins

"Fish is brain food. It is true in terms of intellect, true in terms of mood and depression, true in terms of concentration and attention. And true for a lifetime — from 2 years before conception to old age."

–Jacqueline Stordy

"Amazingly; although the brain constitutes only about 2 percent of body weight, but it can consume upto 20 to 30 percent of the body's entire energy."

–Jean Carper

"You can create more connections—synapses, dendrites and receptors—through diet, supplements, and mental and physical activity. Even adult brain can grow new neurons!"

—Jean Carper

"The ability of a meal's composition to affect the production of brain chemicals distinguishes the brain from all other organs. The crucial compounds that regulate other organs are largely independent of whatever was in the last meal we ate – but not the brain."

—Richard Wurtman

"Simply running a few days a week increases brain proteins, and that helps protect nerve cells from injury, cells known to be associated with cognition."

—Carl Cotman

"The brain is the fattiest organ of our body. The type of fat you put in your brain from birth to death is one of the most critical decisions you can ever make for the good or detriment of your brain."

—Jean Carper

"Don't let omega-6 fats dominate your brain cells. They dispatch assassins that cripple and kill your brain cells, leaving your mental capabilities compromised. You should cut back on omega-6 fats in your diet and eat brain-friendly omega-3 fish oils."

—Shlomo Yehuda

"Omega-3 fats are most fluid fats for keeping cell membranes soft and pliable. While animal fats make cell membranes more crystalline and rigid."

—Hibbelin

"To save your brain from disintegration, you need to eat lots of berries, spinach and other deeply colored fruits and vegetables with high antioxidant activity."

—James A. Joseph

"The genes are the bricks and mortar to build a brain. The environment is the architect."

–Christine Hohmann

"We use only 5% of our intelligence while Albert Einstein used up to 15–20%. There is such a gap between what we do and what we can do."

–William James

"A man who reads too much and uses his own brain too little, falls into lazy habit of thinking."

–Albert Einstein

3

Child Health and Development

"We are guilty of many errors and many faults. But our worst crime is abandoning the children, neglecting the foundation of life. Many of the things we need can wait, the child cannot. Right now is the time his bones and flesh are being formed, his blood is being made. And his senses are being developed. To him we cannot answer tomorrow, his name is TODAY."

—Gabriela Mistral

"I wish you could realize that the destiny of our beloved land lies not with us but in our children."

—Mahatma Gandhi

"Children have more need of role models than of critics."

—Joseph Jonbert

"I do not love him because he is good, but because he is my child."

—Rabindranath Tagore

"When I approach a child, he inspires in me two sentiments, tenderness for what he is, and respect for what he may become."

—Louis Pasteur

"The child is father of the man."

—William Wordsworth

"The true test of a civilization is how well it protects its vulnerable and how well it safeguards its future. Children are both its vulnerable and its future."

—The State of the World's Children, UNICEF 1989

"Children are our most valuable resource."

–Herbert Hoover

"Never have children, only grandchildren."

–Gore Vidal

"It is time to begin attending to the needs and rights of children not as a mere byproduct of progress, but as an end and a means of progress itself."

–The State of the World's Children, UNICEF 1989

"At this moment many millions of children are growing up in circumstances which mean that they will never fulfill the mental and physical potential with which they were born."

–The State of the World's Children, UNICEF 2000

"Parents influence their offsprings eugenically before conception, physiologically during pregnancy and socially after birth. Mother's contribution is far greater than father's."

–RC Mitchell

"The education of the child begins with conception."

–Mahatma Gandhi

"Every child comes with a message that God is not yet discouraged of man."

–Rabindranath Tagore

"Unless you become little children, you cannot know the meaning of life. Children have no knowledge of past and no fear of future, they live in the present moment."

–Jesus

"A boy is of all wild beasts, the most difficult to manage."

–Plato

"Every baby born into the world is finer one than the last."

–Charles Dickens

"Great is the man who has not lost his childlike heart."

—Mencius

"It is a wise father that knows his own child."

—William Shakespeare

"Eighteen goddess like daughters are not equal to one son with a hump."

—Chinese Proverb

"Never threaten children, either punish them or forgive them."

—Talmud

"The prevailing sense of despair at the birth of a female child should be replaced by the awareness and hope that she is the creator and sustainer of progeny."

—Meharban Singh

"The child is a barometer of the family's emotional climate. Behavior and psychological problems in children are a reflection of inter-parental marital conflicts..."

—John Apley

"Before I got married, I had six theories about bringing up children, now I have six children and no theories."

—John Wilmot

"We are aware of the prevailing realities and what we need is to launch a sustained, determined and united crusade to uplift the plight of mothers and their children today because tomorrow may be too late."

—Meharban Singh

"Children are the future of the nation."

—Jawaharlal Nehru

"Newborn is a "blank page" on which environment and education write this or that story of the individual's life."

–J J Rousseau

"The child should be treated as an independent being, a person in his own right, not just your possession. Love him but never possess the child!"

–Anonymous

"Children (especially grandchildren) are the greatest source of fun, joy and celebration in the present and they are our greatest asset and hope for the future."

–Meharban Singh

"The short stature of adults in developing countries is largely due to poor physical growth during the first 3 years of life."

–UN Subcommittee on Nutrition

"An honest man is always a child."

–Socrates

"We constantly discipline our children throughout the day with negative commands—'don't do this', 'don't do that', 'don't jump'—without any positive commands as to 'what actually they should do'. No wonder their subconscious or core is corroded with negative vibes."

–Meharban Singh

"The tragedy is that most parents do love their children, but somehow don't know how to express it in ways that help the child feeling valued, respected and loved."

–Rex Johnson

"When a child is taken to pieces for study, somebody must remember to put the pieces together again."

–John Apley

"If children live with criticism, they learn to condemn.

If children live with hostility, they learn to fight.

If children live with fear, they learn to be apprehensive.

If children live with pity, they learn to feel sorry for themselves.

If children live with ridicule, they learn to be shy.

If children live with jealousy, they learn what envy is.

If children live with shame, they learn to feel guilty.

If children live with tolerance, they learn to be patient.

If children live with praise, they learn to appreciate.

If children live with approval, they learn to like themselves.

If children live with acceptance, they learn to find love in the world.

If children live with recognition, they learn to have a goal.

If children live with sharing, they learn to be generous.

If children live with honesty and fairness, they learn what truth and justice're.

If children live with security, they learn to have faith in themselves and those around them...."

–Dorothy L. Nolte

"Children are not merely small adults and to understand children it is not enough to extrapolate from adults."

—John Apley

"Children seldom misquote you. In fact, they usually repeat word for word what you shouldn't have said."

—John Apley

"Children need your presence more than your presents."

—Jesse Jackson

"The seeds of integrity, character and discipline are sown in childhood. They are planted by parents and tilled by the teachers."

—Meharban Singh

"So long as little children are allowed to suffer, there is no true love in this world."

—Isadora Duncan

"If there is anything that we wish to change in the child, we should first examine it and see whether it is not something that could better be changed in ourselves."

—Carl Jung Gustav

"We recognize that in addition to our separate responsibilities to our individual societies, we have a collective responsibility to uphold the principles of human dignity, equality and equity at the global level. As leaders we have a duty, therefore, to all the world's people, specially the most vulnerable and, in particular, the children of the world, to whom the future belongs."

—UN Millennium Declaration

"Children begin by loving their parents, as they grow older they judge them; rarely, if ever, do they forgive them."

—Oscar Wilde

"The best way to make children good is to make them happy."

—*Oscar Wilde*

"The reason grandparents and grandchildren get along so well is that they have a common enemy."

—*Sam Levenson*

"Adam and Eve had many advantages but the principal one was, that they escaped teething."

—*Mark Twain*

"Spare the rod and spoil the child."

—*English Proverb*

"If you want to give your child only one gift, let it be enthusiasm."

—*Bruce Barton*

Communication and Clinical Examination

4

"Oh God let my mind be ever clean and enlightened. By the bedside of the patient, let no alien thoughts deflect it. Let everything that experience and scholarship have taught, it be present in it and hinder it not in its tranquil work. For great and noble are those scientific judgements that serve the purpose of preserving health and lives of thy creatures........"

–Moimonides bin Musa

"The doctor may learn more about the illness from the way the patient tells the story than from the story itself."

–James B. Herrick

"A great part, I believe, of the art of medicine is the ability to observe. Leave nothing to chance. Overlook nothing, combine contradictory observations and allow yourself enough time."

–Hippocrates

"No observation, however, small or apparently trivial, which fails to fit into a tentative diagnosis, should be put aside as unimportant."

–Henry Cohen

"We have two ears and one tongue so that we would listen more and talk less."

–Diogenese

"Eyes, ears, nose and palpating fingers are the gems of a physician, intact brain is the necklace!"

–Hippocrates

"To study the phenomenon of disease without books is to sail on uncharted sea, while to study books without patients is not to go to the sea at all......"

–William Osler

"Most errors in clinical medicine are made by making a cursory, incomplete examination and not due to lack of knowledge and skills."

–Henry Cohen

"There is only one cardinal rule of medicine, one must always listen to the patient."

–Oliver Sacks

"A doctor who cannot take a good history and a patient who cannot give one, are in danger of giving and receiving bad treatment."

–Anonymous

"There are no short cuts to physical diagnosis. It is learnt only by practice, not a dull and dreary or monotonous practice but practice with all the five senses alert."

–Robert Hutchison

"Observation is the key attribute of a good diagnostician. Keep your eyes and ears open (and mouth shut!)– and be aware, alert and alive with an analytical mind."

–Meharban Singh

"Methods of physicians are like those of a detective, one seeking to explain a disease, other a crime."

–Anonymous

"A person may have learnt very great deal and still be an exceedingly unskillful physician who awakens little confidence in his powers........ . The manner of dealing with patients, of winning their confidence, the art of soothing and consoling them or of drawing their attention to serious matters....... . All this cannot be learnt from the books......"

–John Apley

"What one knows, he sees and what one looks for, he is more likely to see. Chance favors only the prepared mind."

–Louis Pasteur

"Observation is not merely the power of seeing, looking or matching. It should evolve and proceed through a carefully directed analytic exercise to shed new light, provide meaningful insight, propose creative solutions or arrive at novel conclusions."

–William Osler

"It is an amazing fact that among millions of people no two human beings are alike. And whenever you meet and interact with people in your day-to-day life, try to identify subtle differences among them (be it their facial features, mannerisms, demeanor, stance, gait, voice) to sharpen your power of observation and improve your visual memory—a great boon for a clever clinician."

–Meharban Singh

"I know of a doctor who never forgets his stethoscope, blood pressure instrument, his percussion hammer when he starts on his rounds in the morning, yet not infrequently he is so absent-minded as to leave at home one and all important instrument – his brain!"

–RC Cabot

"Doctors record patient's medical history without paying much attention to the patient. But we must never forget that the look on the patient's face, the tremble in his hands, the falter in his speech, the dreams he has, the drawings he makes, are all potential signs (windows) of what really troubles him."

—William Osler

"There is nothing criminal about the student's use of the stethoscope as a status symbol but your status will suffer if your symbol lets you down. Admittedly, the most important part of the stethoscope is the part between the ears – your brain!"

—John Apley

"Symptoms in reality are nothing but cries from suffering body organs."

—Jean-Martin Charcot

"We have two ears and one mouth so that we can listen twice as much as we speak."

—Epictetus

"The most essential part of a student's instruction is obtained not in the lecture-room, but at the bedside. Nothing seen there is lost; the rhythms of disease are learned by frequent repetition; its unforeseen occurrences stamp themselves indelibly in the memory."

—Oliver Wendell Holmes

"We must not explore the chest by percussing our ideas into it. We must rather give our attention to listening to what comes out."

—Friedrich Muller

"Hearing is one of the body's five senses. But listening is an art."

—Frank Tyger

"Never trust a naked male baby; he can shoot without a warning."

–Meharban Singh

"......Illness doesn't strike randomly like a thief in the night. Certain types of people at certain points in their lives will come down with certain kind of ailments......"

–Lisa Alther

"Symptoms are the body's mother tongue, signs are in a foreign language."

–John Brown

"There is no more difficult art to acquire than the art of observation, and for some men it is quite as difficult to record an observation in brief and plain language."

–William Osler

"The important thing is to make the lesson of each case tell on your education. The value of experience is not in seeing much, but in seeing wisely."

–William Osler

"Learn to see, learn to hear, learn to feel, learn to smell, and know that by practice alone can you become expert. Medicine is learned by the bedside and not in the classroom. Let not your conceptions of the manifestations of disease come from words heard in the lecture room or read from the book. See, and then reason and compare and control. But see first."

–William Osler

"Always note and record the unusual. Keep and compare your observations. Communicate or publish short notes on anything that is striking or new."

–William Osler

"All pain is either severe or slight. If slight it is easily endured; if severe it will without doubt be brief."

—Cicero

"Patients must be handled with utmost care and reverence as they are the real books of physicians."

—Meharban Singh

"Don't touch the patient—state first what you see; cultivate your powers of observation."

—William Osler

"Half of us are blind, few of us feel, and we are all deaf."

—William Osler

"The chief function of the consultant is to make a rectal examination that you have omitted."

—William Osler

"Observe, record, tabulate, communicate. Use your five senses."

—William Osler

"One finger in the throat and one in the rectum, makes a good diagnostician."

—William Osler

"The best teaching is that taught by the patient himself."

—William Osler

"The student begins with the patient, continues with the patient, and ends his studies with the patient, using books and lectures as tools, as means to an end."

—William Osler

"The further away the chronic abdominal pain in a child is from the umbilicus, it is more likely to have an organic cause."

—John Apley

"I wish I had time to speak of the value of note-taking. You can do nothing as a student in practice without it. Carry a small notebook which will fit into your waistcoat pocket, and never ask a new patient a question without notebook and pencil in hand."

–William Osler

"In taking histories follow each line of thought; ask no leading questions; never suggest. Give the patient's own words in recording the complaint."

–William Osler

"The four points of a medical student's compass are: Inspection, Palpation, Percussion and Auscultation."

–William Osler

Complementary and Alternative Medicine

5

"The principles of Ayurveda are based on *panchamahabhut* (the five basic elements, i.e. water, earth, fire, air and aether) and the three *doshas* or primary forces, e.g. *prana* or *vata* (air), *agni* or *pitta* (fire) and *soma* or *kapha* or phlegm (water and earth)."

—Rigveda (4000 BC)

"Rather than viewing alternative medicine as a foe to be conquered, a physician would do well to use it to his or her advantage. Even if an alternative treatment hasn't been sufficiently demonstrated to help, it still enables a physician to involve the patient in the healing process."

—Alan Bryson

"Yoga literally yokes or unites body with mind and universal spirit. Yoga places great emphasis on the art of controlled breathing because breathing is the key to control *prana* or the life force."

—Anonymous

"*Alternative medicine*: Set of practices which cannot be tested, refuse to be tested, or consistently fail tests. If a healing technique is demonstrated to have curative properties in properly controlled double-blind trials, it ceases to be alternative. It simply...... becomes medicine."

—Richard Dawkins

"Yoga brings suppleness in body, calmness in mind, kindness in heart and awareness in life."

—Amit Ray

"I believe there are many ways to communicate with your inner self. Words, music, feelings, relaxation, yoga, meditation, hypnotic trance, visualization and prayer can all help you find your way home."

—Bernie Siegel

"Exercise is like prose, whereas yoga is the poetry of movements."

—Amit Ray

"Health is wealth. Peace of mind is happiness. Yoga shows the way."

—Swami Vishnu-Devananda

"The word yoga literally means to join up, or to yoke together. What we're trying to join together in yoga is body, mind and spirit."

—Alison Donley

"Yoga is the practice of quieting the mind."

—Patanjali

"The public has turned to complementary medicine as refugees from the inadequacies of conventional medicine."

—Stephen Fulder

"Relaxation or 'tuning' with one's inner self is associated with Alpha state of brain activity which has profound health benefits—peace of mind, enhanced energy and vitality, improved digestion, lowered blood pressure and slower heart rate, improved immune system, more creativity and better poise and sleep."

—Bernie Siegel

"The formula you need for all the health, success, achievement, wealth and peace of mind, indeed for all the answers to your problems, and I mean all is SSS—Silence, Stillness and Solitude."

—Ron Holland

"An enormous mass of experience, both of homeopathic doctors and their patients, is invoked in favor of the efficacy of these remedies and doses. But the regular profession stands firm in its belief that such experience is worthless and the whole history is one of quackery and delusion."

—William James

"Ayurveda literally means a knowledge of life. It is almost 5000 years old art and science of healing, a way of life, happy and healthy living. Ayurveda adds not only years to life but also life to years."

—Charaka Samhita

"Reiki comes from two Japanese words, Rei and Ki. Rei represents the spiritual source of the universe or higher mind, higher consciousness or divine consciousness. Ki or *chi* in Chinese or *prana* in Sanskrit is a life force energy or divine energy which is free of any negativity. It has the qualities of love, peace, wisdom, compassion and truth. Reiki can thus be defined as spiritually guided life force energy or divine healing power which goes beyond space and time."

—Anonymous

"A positive magnetic field can function like an antibiotic in helping to destroy bacterial, fungal and viral infections by promoting oxygenation and lowering the body's acidity."

—William H. Philpott

"The object of massage is to dispose the effete matters found in the muscles and not expelled by exercise."

—Avicenna

"Therapeutic touch is a contemporary interpretation of several ancient healing practices in which the practitioners consciously direct or sensitively modulate human energies."

–Dolores Krieger

"Fight like with like."

–Samuel Friedrich Hahnemann

"Diseases are orchestrated by asynergy or imbalance between five body elements (*prithvi, soma, agni, vayu* and *akasha*), six *rasas* (sweet, salty, sour, pungent, bitter and astringent), three body humors or constitution (*vata, pitta,* and *kapha*) and three mind doshas (*tamas, rajas,* and *sattva*).

–Ayurvedic doctrine

"The first question an Ayurvedic physician asks is not 'What disease does my patient has?' but 'Who is my patient?' By 'who', the physician does not mean your name, but how you are constituted."

–Deepak Chopra

"Eventually, patients should be able to use their feedback experience to lower their own heart rate or blood pressure, or to alleviate physical complaint. It's a form of self-medication."

–David Spiegel

"Disease is the result of a disruption of the spontaneous flow of nature's intelligence within our physiology. When we violate nature's law and cannot adequately rid ourselves of the results of this disruption, then we have disease."

–Virender Sodhi

"The self-regulation skills acquired through biofeedback training are retained by the individual even after the feedback device is dispensed with."

–Patricia Norris

"Chiropractice embraces the science of life, the knowledge of how organisms act in health and disease and also the art of adjusting the neuroskeleton."

—Daniel David Palmer

"People can see the premature wear and tear in their car's tyres that occurs if the wheels are mal-aligned, yet the same holds true for the human body if the spine is misaligned."

—Robert Blaich

"You may honestly feel grateful that Homeopathy survived the attempts of the Allopaths (orthodoxy) to destroy it."

—Mark Twain

"There is evidence that acupuncture influences production and distribution of a great many neurotransmitters and neuro-modulators, and that in turn alters the perception of pain."

—Maoshing Ni

"Every drug of choice has a receptor site mechanism that is very specific. What we do is to meet the needs of that receptor site by supplying and directing the endorphins and enkephalins through acupuncture."

—Jay Holder

"The essential oils work in a different way than antibiotics, they do not have the usual side effects, and they tend to stimulate the immune system."

—Robert Tisserand

"For many common infectious diseases, aromatherapy offers more effective and more wholesome solution than conventional medicine."

—Kurt Schnaubelt

"Even if conventional medicine tells you that your condition is incurable or that your only option is to live a life dependent on drugs with troublesome side effects, there is hope for improving or reversing your condition by alternative means."

—Leon Chaitow

"The highest ideal of cure is the speedy, gentle and enduring restoration of health by the most trustworthy and least harmful way."

—Samuel Hahnemann

"We now have a separate department of Indian System of Medicine and Homeopathy (ISM and H) which is based on herbal medicines and drugless therapies to combat diseases for which Allopathy has no cure...... India could be a front runner in making the rest of the world aware about the potential of these alternative systems."

—JS Bajaj

"Yoga has a sly, clever way of short-circuiting the mental patterns that cause anxiety."

—Leonardo da Vinci

"There is no alternative medicine. There is only medicine that works and medicine that doesn't work."

—Richard Dawkins

"Every effective drug provokes in the human body a sort of disease of its own and stronger the drug, the more characteristic, and the more marked and violent the disease. We should imitate nature, which sometimes cures a chronic affliction with another supervening disease, and prescribe for the illness we wish to cure, especially if chronic, a drug with power to provoke another, artificial disease, as similar as possible, and the former disease will be cured: *fight like with like.*"

—Samuel Hahnemann

"There is a need for integrated system of health care delivery in India, optimally functional with contributions of all health care providers including allied health professionals and physicians from all systems of medicine, at all levels of primary, secondary and tertiary health care."

–JS Bajaj

"Molecular biology and molecular pharmacology provide a new interface between Ayurveda and modern medicine, since the Ayurvedic concepts of *vata, pitta* and *kapha* are essentially concepts of molecular biology."

–RD Lele

6

Death and Dying

"Death should not be viewed as a tragedy but a peaceful acceptance, a loving entry into the unknown, a blissful acceptance of ultimate truth and joyful goodbye to all friends and foes."

–Bhagvad Gita

"Death may be the greatest of all human blessings."

–Socrates

"He whom the gods favor, dies in youth."

–Plautus

"We all labor against our own cure, for death is the cure of all diseases."

–Thomas Browne

"Death is the golden key that opens the palace of eternity."

–Milton

"The fear of death is worse than death."

–Robert Burton

"*Vaidyaraja namas thubhyam yamaraja sahodharam Yamena harati pranath vaidaha pranani dhanani cha!*"

–Sanskrit Shloka

(Oh, doctor I salute you. You are just like Yamaraja, the god of death. While Yamaraja takes away life, you take away the patient's life as well as his money)

"Whom the gods love dies young."

—*Menander*

"Death is a punishment to some, to some a gift, and to many a favor."

—*Seneca*

"When you were born, you cried and the world rejoiced. Live your life in such a manner that when you die, the world cries and you rejoice."

—*Indian Saying*

"Well now, there's a remedy for everything except death."

—*Cervantes*

"When fate arrives, the physician becomes a fool."

—*Arabic Proverb*

"Nothing in life is certain except death and taxes."

—*Benjamin Franklin*

"If you can love death, you become deathless... If you can love non-being then nothing can destroy you, you have transcended time and space."

—*Osho*

"Death and taxes and childbirth! There's never any convenient time for any of them."

—*Margaret Mitchell*

"A man is not completely born until he is dead."

—*Benjamin Franklin*

"Death is not the greatest loss in life. The greatest loss is what dies while we live."

—*Norman Cousins*

"Death is only the beginning..."

—Imhotep

"Death borders upon our birth, and our cradle stands in the grave. Our birth is nothing but our death begun."

—Bishop Hall

"Fear not the death, for the sooner we die, the longer we shall be immortal."

—Benjamin Franklin

"By medicine life may be prolonged, yet death will seize the doctor too."

—William Shakespeare

"A good man never dies."

—Callimachus

"Death is the ultimate paradise for peace. Every one will reach this stage sooner or later—no one can escape the ultimate truth."

—Kandasamy Rangarajan

"The goal of life is death."

—Sigmund Freud

"To desire immortality is to desire the eternal perpetuation of a great mistake."

—Schopenhauer

"Despite all the technological advances, medicine can never achieve immortality—death is more certain than birth."

—Meharban Singh

"Birth is messenger of death."

—Syrian Proverb

"Eat, drink and be merry, for tomorrow we shall die."
—Imhotep

"We don't know life, how can me know death?"
—Confucius

"From dust thou art and unto dust shalt thou return."
—Old Testament

"Wonderful is the courage that conquers death."
—Jawaharlal Nehru

"Cast off the fear of death from your heart and live a full life."
—Rigveda

"Death is the greatest truth of life. It is because we fear death so much for ourselves that we shed tears over the death of others."
—Mahatma Gandhi

"Death does not concern us, because as long as we exist, death is not here. And when it does come, we no longer exist."
—Epicurus

"Life is pleasant, death is peaceful. It's the transition that's troublesome."
—Isaac Asimov

"It is as natural to die, as to be born."
—Bacon

"Death is poor man's doctor."
—Irish Proverb

"The good die first."
—William Wordsworth

"Birth and death are not two different states, but they are different aspects of the same state."

—Mahatma Gandhi

"The human body is a furnace which keeps in blast three score years and ten, more or less...... when the fire slackens, life declines, when it goes out, we are dead."

—Oliver Wendell Holmes

"Death is not extinguishing the light, it is putting out the lamp because dawn has come."

—Rabindranath Tagore

"Men fear death as children fear to go in the dark and as that natural fear in children is increased with tales, so is the other."

—Francis Bacon

"Most people are not afraid of death but are scared of mode of dying. The blessed one's die in sleep and in peace."

—Meharban Singh

"Death is a solemn experience, a change from which no one can escape. One who does not prepare for it is a fool."

—Swami Rama

"Celebrate while you are alone and celebrate when you are with people. Celebrate silence and celebrate noise, celebrate life and celebrate death."

—Francois Gautier

"It was in the darkness that I found light. It was in the pain that I found the gain. It was in the dying that I found the life. It was in aloneness that I found the need of prayer. And it is through the love of God that I found meaning in my life. I have thus finally learnt that it is through the loss of anykind, that there is something worthwhile or of a greater dimension to be gained."

—Susan Duffy

"Everyone dies. But not everyone really lives."

—William Wallace

"When fate arrives, the physician becomes a fool."

—Arabic Proverb

"The body is not a permanent dwelling, but a sort of inn which is to be left behind when one perceives that one is a burden to the host."

—Seneca

"There is no cure for birth and death save to enjoy the interval."

—George Santayana

"We avoid being with our patients in their last moments because we see their death as our failure. When we realize that our role is to heal, and not to stop death, then we will understand what an honor it can be to share a person's last moments."

—Anonymous

"There are worse things in life than death. Have you ever spent an evening with an insurance salesman?"

—Woody Allen

"People have wrong idea about death. They see it as an end, but it is really a beginning."

—Maharishi Mahesh Yogi

"Let us endeavor to live such a life that when we come to die even the undertaker will be sorry."

—Mark Twain

"It is not the death or pain that is to be dreaded, but the fear of pain or death."

—Epictetus

"*Vaidayo Yama Sahodaraha*—The doctor is the elder brother of the God of death—Yama"

—*Indian Saying*

"The difficulty is not in avoiding death, but in avoiding unrighteousness, for it runs faster than death."

—*Socrates*

"Oh Death, the poor man's dearest friend...... The kindest and the best."

—*Robert Burns*

"Why is it that we rejoice at birth and grieve at a funeral? Is it because we are not the person concerned?"

—*Mark Twain*

"I believe it should be possible for someone striken with a serious and ultimately fatal illness to choose to die peacefully with medical help, rather than suffer."

—*Terry Pratchett*

"I have careful records of about five hundred death-beds...... Ninety suffered bodily pain or distress of one kind or another, eleven showed mental apprehension, two positive terror, one expressed spiritual exaltation, one bitter remorse. The great majority gave no sign one way or the other; like their birth their death was asleep and a forgetting."

—*William Osler*

"Death is not the worse that can happen to men."

—*Plato*

"Fear of death is the most unjustified of all fears, for there's no risk of accident for someone who's dead."

—*Albert Einstein*

"To know life, one has to learn the art of dying. Those who die consciously with awareness and a welcoming heart, the death disappears and it becomes a door to a state of death-lessness, the eternal awakening."

—Upanishads

"Death is certain for the born, and rebirth is inevitable for the dead. You should not, therefore, grieve over the inevitable."

—Bhagavad Gita

"Celebrate birth, celebrate life, celebrate death. Death is divine because that indeed is the very culmination of life."

—Osho

"When death is near, neither doctors nor medicines help."

—Sicilian Proverb

7

Diet, Nutrition and Fasting

"No illness that can be treated by diet should be treated by any other means."

—Maimonides bin Musa

"Let thy food be thy medicine and thy medicine be thy food."

—Hippocrates

"Most of us are over-fed and undernourished. We suffer from obesity and malnutrition at the same time because our foods are nutritionally depleted."

—Mike Adams

"Food is the breakthrough drug of the 21st century."

—Jean Carper

"Vitamins should be seen as supplements and not as substitutes for a well-balanced diet."

—Alan Bryson

"As long as man continues to be ruthless destroyer of lower living beings, he will never know health or peace. For as long as men massacre animals, they will kill each other."

—Pythagoras

"If your diet is wrong, no medicine can help; If your diet is correct, you won't need any medicine."

—Victor G. Rocine

"To extend your life by a year, take one less bite each meal."
—Chinese Proverb

"Our bodies need food to keep us healthy and our souls need love to grow."
—Master Ching Hai

"When you're green inside, you're clean inside."
—Bernard Jensen

"The best of all medicines are rest and fasting."
—Benjamin Franklin

"One who takes medicines and neglects his diet, wastes the skills of his physician."
—Chinese Proverb

"Drinking water is like taking a shower inside, it is a cleansing operation."
—Alan Bryson

"Do not neglect medical treatment when it is necessary, but leave it off when health has been restored. Treat disease through diet, by preference, refraining from the use of drugs…"
—Baha'ullah

"Fish to taste fine must swim three times—in the water, in oil and in wine."
—Polish Proverb

"We are basically vegetarian species and should be eating a wide variety of plant foods and minimising our intake of animal foods."
—T. Colin Campbell

"The time will come when meat will no longer be eaten. Medical science is only in its infancy, yet it has shown that our natural food is that which grows out of the ground…

When mankind is more fully developed, the eating of meat will gradually cease."

—Abdul-Bahá

"Cater to your hunger and not to your appetite, fulfill it with nourishing food and not through junky cravings. Man seeks to change natural foods to suit his taste, thereby putting an end to the very essence of life contained in them."

—Sathya Sai Baba

"By eating meat, if you wish to make your body a graveyard that's your prerogative, but please respect my right not to do so."

—Anonymous

"Pediatricians eat because children don't ......"

—John Apley

"One should eat to live, not live to eat."

—Cicero

"More people have been killed by overeating and drinking than by the sword."

—William Osler

"Besides agreeing with the aims of vegetarianism for aesthetic and moral reasons, it is my view that a vegetarian manner of living by its purely physical effect on the human temperament would most beneficially influence the lot of mankind."

—Albert Einstein

"We are what we eat."

—Ludwig Feuerbach

"Most children hate two things; eating green leafy vegetables and drinking milk. When parents are more concerned about a food item, children are least interested—they virtually blackmail their parents."

—Meharban Singh

"Vegetarianism is harmless, although it is apt to fill a man with wind and self-righteousness."

—Robert Hutchison

"Today, more than 95% of all chronic diseases are caused by faulty food choice, toxic food ingredients, nutritional deficiencies and lack of physical exercise."

—Mike Adams

"Japanese key to health is *hara a bachi bu*—which means that "Your stomach at eight-tenths you won't need a doctor." The best mantra for longevity is "stop eating when you're 80% full."

—Japanese Saying

"A very important factor in obesity is overeating, a vice which is more prevalent and only a little behind overdrinking in its disastrous effects. A majority of persons over forty years of age habitually eat too much."

—William Osler

"No diet will ever remove all the fat from your body because the brain is entirely fat."

—George Bernard Shaw

"Most people dig their own graves with their knives and forks."

—Parmahansa Yoganand

"In eating, a third of the stomach should be filled with food, a third with drink and the rest left empty."

—Talmud

"In general, since the improvement of cookery, mankind eat twice as much as nature requires."

—Benjamin Franklin

"The best way to make a child eat is not to try."

—Meharban Singh

"More people die in the United States of too much food than of too little."

—John Kenneth Galbraith

"One-quarter of what you eat keeps you alive. The three-quarters keeps your doctor alive."

—Egyptian Proverb

"Eat breakfast like a king, lunch like a prince and dinner like a pauper."

—Popular Saying

"Men live to eat, while I eat to live."

—Socrates

"One cannot think well, love well, sleep well, if one has not dined well."

—Virginia Woolf

"Eat to live, don't live to eat."

—Benjamin Franklin

"Lunch kills half of Paris, supper the other half."

—Montesquieu

"When diet is wrong, medicine is of no use. When diet is correct, there is no need for any medicine."

—Ayurvedic Proverb

"You become what you eat! Food we eat influence our memory, comprehension, thinking, judgement, intellect and emotions."

—Anonymous

"To save your brain from disintegration, you need to eat lots of berries, spinach and other deeply colored fruits and vegetables with high antioxidant activity."

—James A. Joseph

"From high fat to low fat with age, first to increase intelligence and then to increase life span!"

—Kurt Widhalm

"Nothing will benefit human health and increase the chances for survival of life on earth as much as the evolution to a vegetarian diet."

—Albert Einstein

"Food that is good for the heart is likely to be good for the brain."

—Hipprocrates

"Leave your drugs in the chemist's pot if you can heal the patient with food."

—Hippocrates

"Let food be your medicine, let medicine be your food."

—Imhotep

"There is compelling evidence to show that breakfast can boost brain functioning—learning, memory, academic performance—and general emotional and psychological wellbeing."

—J. Michael Murphy

"Butter is gold in the morning, silver at noon, lead at night."

—Popular Saying

"The doctor of the future will no longer treat the human frame with drugs, but rather will care and prevent disease with nutrition."

—Thomas Edison

"The human body heals itself and nutrition provides the resources to accomplish the task."

–Roger Williams

"Eating white potatoes or white bread is just like eating candy, as far as body knows."

–Walter Willett

"Infant feeding, a subject that upon superficial thought seems so simple that the majority of medical students are apt to pass it by as pertaining to the nurse and not the doctor."

–JM Keating

"Fruits are the most spiritually beneficial of all foods."

–Parmahansa Yogananda

"After dinner sit a while, after supper walk a mile."

–Popular Saying

"Enjoy and feel every bite of food and every sip of liquid you take. You must visualize that food and drinks are not only satisfying your hunger and thirst but are also generating health in your body and mind."

–Buddha

"Human beings are supposed to live more than a hundred and fifty years. But we eat in a way that immediately begins to destroy us. Diets that create the acidic milieu starts the process of invasion by microbes and suppress our vibrational energy level."

–James Redfield

"Feeding the sick is the greatest of all virtues."

–Indian Proverb

"Dieting is a system of starving yourself to death so that you can live a little longer."

–Jan Murray

"Bad men live to eat and drink; whereas good men eat and drink in order to live."

–Socrates

"An apple a day, keeps the doctor away."

–English Proverb

"Cow's milk protein may be the single most significant carcinogen to which humans are exposed."

–T. Colin Campbell

"A pomegranate a day, keeps the cardiologist away."

–Author Unknown

"Could you look an animal in the eyes and say to it, "My appetite is more important than your suffering."

–Moby

"For as long as men massacre animals, they will kill each other. Indeed, he who sows, the seeds of murder and pain, cannot reap joy and love.

–Pythogoras

"In every 10 seconds we lose a child to hunger. This is more than HIV/AIDS, malaria and tuberculosis combined."

–Josette Sheeran

"The secret of longevity is to have a very good breakfast, to share lunch with one's friends and give the dinner to your enemy."

–Chinese Proverb

"I never worry about diets. The only "carrots" that interest me are those you get in a diamond."

–Andy Warhol

"Give a man a fish, and you feed him for one day. Teach him how to fish, and you feed him for a life time."

—Lao Tzu

"Eating fruits and vegetables is better than taking a vitamin pill."

—Rui Hai Liu

"If you want to live a healthy and active life, drink whey. And if everyone was raised on whey, doctors would be bankrupt."

—Italian Proverb

"Health requires healthy food."

—Roger Williams

"The absorption and organization of sunlight, the essence of life, is derived almost exclusively through plants. Since light is the driving force of every cell in our bodies, that is why we need green plants."

—Bircher Benner

"To lengthen thy life, lessen thy meals."

—Benjamin Franklin

"If a child in his first 1000 days—from conception to two years old—does not have adequate nutrition, the damage is irreversible."

—Josette Sheeran

"Fasting is the first principle of medicine."

—Jalaluddin Rumi

"Fasting is an effective and safe method of detoxifying the body—a technique that wise men have used for centuries to heal the sick. Fast regularly and help the body heal itself and stay well."

—James Balch

"Fasting cleanses the soul, raises the mind, subjects one's flesh to the spirit, renders the heart contrite and humble, scatters the clouds of concupiscence, quenches the fire of lust, and kindles the true light of chastity."

—St. Augustine

"One who believes, fasting is prescribed for you… as it was prescribed for those before you, so that you may safeguard yourselves against every kind of ill and become righteous."

—Quran

"Fasting is a natural method of healing."

—Paramahansa Yogananda

"A man can live and be healthy without killing animals for food; therefore, if he eats meat, he participates in taking animal life merely for the sake of his appetite. And to act so is immoral."

—Leo Tolstoy

"I choose not to make a graveyard of my body for the rotting corpses of dead animals."

—George Bernard Shaw

"Although man has included meat in his diet for thousand of years, his anatomy, physiology and chemistry of his digestive juices, are still unmistakably those of a frugivorous animal."

—Herbert M. Shelton

"Soft drinks are loaded with ingredients and toxins which are credited to cause a host of health problems like caries of teeth, acidity, gastro-esophageal reflux, obesity, osteoporosis, allergic disorders, neurotoxicity, restlessness and addiction. There is a need to print a statutary warning:

"Excessive intake of soft drinks is hazardous to the health of children."

—Meharban Singh

"O, thou beautiful damsel, may the four oceans of the earth contribute the secretion of milk in thy breasts for the purpose of improving the bodily strength of the child. O, thou with the beautiful face, may child reared on your milk, attain a long life, like the gods made immortal with drinks of nectar.

—Sushruta Samhita

"My best performances were when I was 30 years old, and I was a vegan."

—Carl Lewis

8

Diseases, Disability and Diagnosis

"There is no such thing as never or always in medicine. The greater the ignorance, the greater would be dogmatism. Medicine is a science of uncertainty and an art of probability."

—William Osler

"Symptoms in reality are nothing but the cry from the suffering organs."

—Jean Martin Charcot

"*Diagnosis*: A physicians' forecast of disease by the patients' pulse and purse."

—Ambrose Bierce

"Disease is nothing else but an attempt on the part of body to rid itself of morbific matter."

—Thomas Sydenham

"Uncommon manifestations of a common disorder are more common than common manifestations of a rare disease."

—Paul Cutler

"If you are hidebound with prejudice, if your temper is sentimental, you can go through the wards of the hospital and be as ignorant a man at the end as you were in the beginning."

—W. Somerset Maugham

"Do germs cause the disease or could it be the other way around...... first the disease then the germs. Most diseases occur when people allow themselves to become enervated, that is, low in nerve energy."

–Alec Burton

"We know a great deal about the causes of disease than we do about the causes of health."

–M. Scott Peck

"Diagnosis is not the end, but the beginning of medical practice."

–Martin H. Fischer

"My advice to other disabled people would be, concentrate on things your disability doesn't prevent you doing well, and don't regret the things it interferes with. Don't be disabled in spirit as well as physically."

–Stephen Hawking

"A true scientist does not set out to prove something, he has to learn to follow where the facts lead him. He should know the art of whipping his prejudices to get pearls."

–Spallanzani

"The doctor may learn more about the illness from the way the patient tells the story than from the story itself."

–James B. Herrick

"If you want to be a good doctor, avoid "bulldozing" a diagnosis...... To indulge in a large number of investigations, or to repeat and extend them without good reason, is both crude medicine and distasteful."

–John Apley

"A smart mother often makes a better diagnosis than a dull doctor."

–August Bier

"Disease is the warning and, therefore, the friend, not the enemy of mankind."

–George S. Weger

"When you are sick of your sickness, you are no longer sick."

–Chinese Proverb

"The greatest of follies is to sacrifice health for any other kind of happiness."

–Schopenhauer

"When making a diagnosis be ambitious. The further your diagnosis goes, the more you will be able to help the patient by extending the scope of treatment or by prevention."

–John Apley

"The fact that your patient gets well does not prove that your diagnosis was correct."

–Samuel J. Meltzer

"All that wheezes is not asthma. Before you attach the asthma label, you should rule out some non-asthmatic causes of wheezing."

–John Apley

"When the cause of a disease is discovered, physicians consider that the cure is discovered."

–Cicero

"Your genome knows much more about your medical history than you do."

–W. Daniel Hillis

"They do certainly give very strange, and newfangled names to diseases."

–Plato

"One CT scan is worth a room full of neurologists."

–Atkinson Morley

"What is impossible to see from the viewpoint of those who believe in cures is that the very symptoms the good doctors have suppressed and turned into chronic disease were the body's only means of correcting the problem! The so called "disease" was the only "cure" possible!"

–Philip Chapman

"Be careful about reading health books. You may die of misprint."

–Mark Twain

"There is no disease more conducive to clinical humility than aneurysm of the aorta."

–William Osler

"First the doctor told me the good news. I was going to have a disease named after me."

–Steve Martin

"To confess ignorance is often wiser than to beat about the bush with a hypothetical diagnosis."

–William Osler

"Absolute diagnoses are unsafe, and are made at the expense of the conscience."

–William Osler

"Where a man feels pain he lays his hand."

–Dutch Proverb

"The greater the ignorance, the greater the dogmatism."

–William Osler

"Start out with the conviction that absolute truth is hard to reach in matters relating to our fellow creatures, healthy or diseased, that slips in observation are inevitable even with the best trained faculties, that errors in judgement must occur in the practice of an art which consists largely in balancing probabilities—start, I say, with this attitude of mind... you will draw from your errors the very lessons which may enable you to avoid their repetition."

—*William Osler*

"The concept of total wellness recognizes that every thought, word and behavior affects our greater health and well being. And we, in turn, are affected not only emotionally but also physically and spiritually."

—*Greg Anderson*

"Pneumonia is the captain of the men of death and tuberculosis is the handmaid."

—*William Osler*

"A patient with a written list of symptoms—neurasthenia."

—*William Osler*

"If you talk to god, you are praying. But if god talks to you, you have schizophrenia."

—*Thomas Szasz*

"It is well to be up before day break, for such a habit contributes to health, wealth and wisdom."

—*Aristotle*

"We need to re-direct our perspectives of microbes and see them in a new light. Bacteria infact assist us in many ways by protecting us from other organisms (like fungi), assisting in digestion and metabolism of food, synthesizing vitamins and helping to eliminate waste materials."

—*Paul Goldberg*

"Hygienists object to the germ theory of disease because germs do not cause disease. They may be present in disease processes and they may complicate a disease with their waste products which can be very toxic at times, but the germ or virus alone is never a sole cause of disease."

–Virginia V. Vetrano

"Germs do not cause disease. Nature never surrounds her children with enemies. It is the individual who invites disease in his own body because of poor living habits. We should remember that germs are friends and scavengers attracted by disease rather than enemies causing disease—the germ theory and vaccination are kept going by commercialism."

–Robert R. Gross

"This day relenting God hath placed within my hand, a wondrous thing; and God be praised. At his command seeking his secret deeds, with tears and toiling breath, I find thy cunning seeds, O million-murdering death. I know this little thing, a myriad men will save. O death, where is thy sting. Thy victory, O grave?

–Ronald Ross

(He wrote this poem following his discovery of malarial parasite in the mosquito)

"Disease is the biggest money maker in our economy."

–John H. Tobe

9

Drugs and Therapeutic Options

"*Prescription*: A physician's guess at what will best prolong the situation with least harm to the patient."
—Ambrose Bierce

"It is easy to get a thousand prescriptions but hard to get one single remedy."
—Chinese Proverb

"During the 1830s...... the common practice of bloodletting was used to treat almost every known ailment. Bleeding did patients no good at best; at worst, it weakened and killed them."
—Science Astray

"The placebo is one of the most powerful medicines we have. It's hard to tell sometimes whether what we're doing is more than the placebo effect."
—Thomas Delbanco

"Drugs are not always necessary. Belief in recovery always is."
—Norman Cousins

"The best doctor gives the least medicine."
—Benjamin Franklin

"Patients demand antibiotics. It takes a minute to write a prescription, but it takes 15–20 minutes not to write a prescription."

—Neil Fishman

"Of all the remedies that has pleased the almighty God to give man to relieve his suffering, none is so universal and so efficacious as opium."

—Thomas Sydenham

"Medicines are the third leading cause of death in United States after heart disease and cancer."

—US Health Statistics

"Nearly all men eventually die of their medicines, and not of their diseases."

—Moliere

"Poisons in small doses are best medicines and useful medicines in too large doses are poisonous."

—Williams Withering

"Anyone who believes that anything can be suited to everyone is a great fool, because medicine is practiced not on mankind in general but on an individual in particular."

—Henri de Mondeville

"When a lot of remedies for a disease are suggested, it generally means it cannot be cured."

—Sushruta

"Most illnesses are cured without the physician's help through the aid of nature. If you can cure the patient by dietary means, do not turn to drugs. Do not rely on cure-alls for they mostly rest on ignorance and superstition."

—Hebrew

"Doctors think that a lot of their patients are cured not knowing that they have simply quit in disgust."

—Don Herold

"Half the modern drugs could well be thrown out of the window, except that there is a fear that birds might eat them."

—Martin H. Fischer

"All who drink of this remedy recover in a short time, except those whom it does not help, who all die. Therefore, it is obvious that it fails only in incurable cases."

—Galen

"Water is the elixir of life; it purifies the body and we become energetic. Water has medicinal value and it frees body from different *doshas* (ailments)."

—Atharva Veda

"A doctor would promise life to a corpse if it could swallow the pills."

—Napolean Bonaparte

"If the whole materia medica as being used now, could be sunk to the bottom of the sea, it would be better for all mankind—but all the worse for the fishes."

—Oliver Wendell Holmes

"Why would a patient swallow poison because he is ill, or take that which would make a well man sick."

—LF Kebbler

"You have a cough? Go home tonight, take a whole box of a laxative—tomorrow you'll be afraid to cough."

—Pearl Williams

"The responsible clinicians must be able to help their patients to go through all the therapeutic options, including those that they may find unconventional because patients increasingly want informed and shared decision making about their health."

—Avrum Bluming

"You may know the intractability of a disease by its long list of remedies."

—Alonzo Clark

"Many dishes, many diseases; many medicines, few cures."

—*Benjamin Franklin*

"Most diseases recover spontaneously and no drug is entirely safe—virtually every drug has side effects including a placebo."

—*Meharban Singh*

"When a lot of remedies are suggested for a disease, that means it cannot be cured."

—*Anton Chekhov*

"I confidently affirm that the greater part of those who are supposed to have died of gout, have died of the medicine rather than the disease."

—*Thomas Sydenham*

"The use of drugs as a first resource leads to neglect of other methods, which may be equally or even more effective. Remember, not everybody needs treatment."

—*John Apley*

"Poisons and medicines are often times the same substance given with different intents."

—*Peter Mere Latham*

"The desire to take medicine is perhaps the greatest feature which distinguishes man from animals."

—*William Osler*

"The physician should have faith in his clinical acumen and should treat the patient and not his laboratory reports."

—*John Apley*

"Walking is man's best medicine."

—*Hippocrates*

"Avoid nostrums and patent medicines. The habitual use of any drug is harmful. The most eminent physicians are now agreed that very few drugs have any real curative value. The essential thing is right habits of life."
                                                    –*John Harvey Kellogg*

"Medicine cures the man, who is fated not to die."
                                                    –*Chinese Proverb*

"Love cures people—both the ones who give it and the ones who receive it."
                                                    –*Karl Meninger*

"Medicine is a collection of uncertain prescriptions, the results of which, taken collectively, are more fatal than useful to mankind."
                                                    –*Napoleon Bonaparte*

"*Similia similibus curentur,* i.e. "like may be cured by like."
                                                    –*Samuel Hahnemann*

"Men worry over the great number of diseases, while doctors worry over the scarcity of effective remedies."
                                                    –*Pien Ch'iao*

"Some remedies are worse than the disease."
                                                    –*Publilius Syrus*

"Doctors prescribe medicines of which they know little, to cure diseases of which they know less, in human beings of which they know nothing."
                                                    –*Voltaire*

"The worst thing about medicine is that one kind makes another necessary."
                                                    –*Elbert Hubbard*

"When will they realize that there are too many drugs? No fewer than 150,000 preparations are now in use. About 15,000 new mixtures and formulations hit the market each year, while about 12,000 medicines die off...... We simply don't have enough diseases to go around. At the moment the most helpful contribution is the new drug to counteract the untoward effect of other new drugs."

–Walter Modell

"Meditation is better than medications for a healthy heart."

–Anonymous

"The medicine may be worse than the malady."

–Francis Beaumont

"The best and most efficient pharmacy is within your own system."

–Robert C. Peale

"Today's medicine is at the end of its road. It can no longer be transformed, modified, readjusted. That's been tried too often. Today's medicine must die in order to be reborn. We must prepare its complete renovation."

–Maurice Delort

"He's the best physician that knows the worthlessness of the most medicines."

–Benjamin Franklin

"Every month, millions are in fact being damaged by treatment which is supposed to be helping them."

–Werner Lehmpfuhl

"I believe that the medical treatments of various abnormal conditions arising in infants, are likely to be dietetic in future, rather than by means of drugs."

–Thomas M. Rotch

"I am dying from the treatment of too many physicians."
—Alexander The Great

"I wonder why ye can always read a doctor's bill, an'ye never can read his prescription."
—Firly Peter Dunne

"The field of western medicine has become literally nothing but "medicine". Doctors are on their way out, to be replaced by self-service pharmaceutical vending machines."
—Grey Livingston

"Why do we pay for psychotherapy when massages cost half as much."
—Jason Love

"Botany, the eldest daughter of medicine."
—Johann Hermann Baas

"Water, air, and cleanliness are the chief articles in my pharmacy."
—Napoleon Bonaparte

"To do nothing is also a good remedy."
—Hippocrates

"To live by medicine is to live horribly."
—Carolus Linnaeus

"It requires a great deal of faith for a man to be cured by his own placebos."
—John L. Meclenahan

"Patients may recover in spite of drugs or because of them."
—JH Gaddum

"In medicine sins of commission are mortal, sins of omission are venial."
—Theodore Tronchin

"There is no curing a sick man who believes himself to be in health."

—Henri Amiel

"Laughter is the best medicine."

—Norman Cousins

"A vigorous five-mile walk will do more good for an unhappy but otherwise healthy adult than all the medicines and psychology in the world."

—Paul Dudley White

"Fever is a friend and not a foe—never try to give it a knocking blow!"

—Meharban Singh

"The public blames the medical profession for giving too many tranquilizers and antidepressants. But what would you do? Doctors like to see healing as a result of their work. Yet today we often must be content with far less. There are so many things wrong with people's lives that even our best is only a stopgap."

—Richard A. Swenson

"One of the first duties of the physician is to educate the masses not to take medicine."

—William Osler

"Dermatology is the only speciality in medicine where there are 200 diseases and only three types of creams to treat them."

—Anonymous

"Medicines heal doubts as well as diseases."

—Karl Marx

"Corticosteroids are the refuge of the therapeutically destitute."

—Anonymous

"The two underlying principles of dermatology: if it is wet then dry it, if it is dry then wet it."
—*Anonymous*

"My opinion is, that more harm than good is done by physicians, and I am convinced, that, had I left my patients to nature, instead of prescribing drugs, more would have been saved."
—*Christoph Wilhelm Hufeland*

"In modern medicine, we have a name for nearly everything, but cure for almost nothing."
—*Charles F. Glassman*

"There is no such thing as incurables, there are only things for which man has not found a cure so far."
—*Bernard M. Baruch*

"The use of 'shotgun' antibiotic therapy is the refuge of an ill experienced physician, who lacks confidence in himself and in his diagnostic skills."
—*Meharban Singh*

"Those diseases which medicines do not cure, iron (the knife) cures, those which iron cannot cure, fire cures; and those which fire cannot cure, are to be reckoned wholly incurable."
—*Hippocrates*

"Prayers promote the process of healing; perhaps doctor in future should prescribe prayers "three times a day" along with their patients' regular treatment."
—*William Nolen*

"The body has its own biological wisdom to heal thyself. The living body is the best pharmacy ever devised. It produces diuretics, painkillers, tranquilizers, sleeping pills, antibiotics, probiotics—indeed everything manufactured by the drug companies. And it makes them much, much better."
—*Deepak Chopra*

"What I call a good patient is one who, having found a good physician, sticks to him till he dies."

–Oliver Wendell Holmes

"Desperate diseases must have desperate cures."

–Popular Saying

"I think that the best kind of medicine is the gentlest treatment that produces the maximum healing response."

–Andrew Weil

"Keep the patient under best conditions like fresh air, sunlight, plentiful space, nutritious food, warmth, clean surroundings, solitude—and allow nature to heal the patient."

–Florence Nightingale

"Yoga is the best medicine to live the life fullest."

–Narendra Modi

"To do nothing is sometimes a good remedy."

–Hippocrates

"The young physician starts life with twenty drugs for each disease, and the old physician ends life with one drug for twenty diseases."

–William Osler

"It is an unfortunate fact that more people in the world are now suffering from drugs and not from diseases. And no drug is entirely safe while most diseases are either mild or self-limiting."

–Meharban Singh

"You can die of the cure, before you die of the disease."

–Michael Landon

"Remember how little you know and how much you do not know. Do not pour strange medicines into your patients."

—William Osler

"But know also, man has an inborn craving for medicines. Generations of heroic dosings have given his tissues such a thirst...for drugs. As I once before remarked, the desire to take medicine is one feature which distinguishes man, the animal, from his fellow creatures. It is really one of the most serious difficulties with which we have to contend. Even in minor ailments, which would yield to dieting or to simple home remedies, the doctor's visit is not thought to be complete without the prescription."

—William Osler

"Medicine sometimes snatches away health, sometimes gives it."

—Ovid

"There are two great medicines; diet and self-control."

—Max Bircher

"He cures most in whom most have faith."

—Galen

"Care more particularly for the individual patient than for the special features of the disease."

—William Osler

"Common cold takes seven days to resolve. But when you treat it, it gets cured in one week."

—Popular Saying

"I find medicine is the best of all trades because whether you do any good or not, you still get your money."

—Moliere

"A man who cannot work without his hypodermic needle is a poor doctor. The amount of narcotic you use is inversely proportional to your skills."

–Martin H. Fischer

"Happiness is the most powerful of all tonics."

–Herbert Spence

"We do know that no two individuals are alike—whether it be in looks, thoughts, actions, emotions, biorhythms, psycho-immuno-neurology axis, enzymic characteristics, metabolic processes, genetic code — so on and so forth. But in modern system of medicine, we prescribe the same medicine, in the same dose, through the same route and for the same duration to every patient which is obviously too simplistic and naïve."

–Meharban Singh

"Treat the patient, not his X-rays."

–James M. Hunter

"You should not poison your body into health with drugs, chemo or radiation. Health can only be achieved with healthful living."

–TC Fry

"Physicians of the utmost fame were called, but when they came they answered as they took fees, "there is no cure for this disease"."

–Hilaire Belloc

"Even if no medicine is necessary, physician should prescribe some harmless concoction, lest the patient thinks the treatment not worth the fee, and lest nature should seem to have healed the patient without the physician's aid."

–Archimatheus

"Sleep is like a drug—if you take it too much at a time, it makes you dopey and you lose time, vitality and opportunities."
—*Thomas Edison*

"Most over-the-counter and almost all prescribed drugs merely mask symptoms or control health problems or in some way alter the way organs or systems work. Drugs almost never deal with the reasons why these problems exist, while they frequently create new health problems as side effects of their activities."
—*John R. Lee*

"Insulin is not a cure for diabetes, it is a treatment. It enables the diabetic to burn sufficient carbohydrates, so that proteins and fats may be added to the diet in sufficient quantities to provide energy for economic burdens of life."
—*Frederick Grant Banting*

"The best of all medicines is resting and fasting."
—*Benjamen Franklin*

"All drugs are poisons, the benefit depends upon dosage."
—*Paracelsus*

"The books we read should be chosen with great care because they are truly "the medicines of the soul"."
—*Oliver Wendell Holmes*

"Medicine makes people ill, mathematics makes them sad, and theology makes them sinful."
—*Martin Luther*

"Words are the most powerful drug used by the mankind."
—*Rudyard Kipling*

"When you are sick, you can call a doctor. But it is more important to call those who love you because there is no medicine more important than love."
—*Osho*

Ethics, Moral Principles and Humanities

"No other gift is greater than the gift of life. The patient may doubt his relatives, his sons and even his parents but he has full faith in his physician. He gives himself up in the doctor's hands and has no misgivings about him, therefore, it is the physician's duty to look after him as his own......"

–Charaka

"What we do not say and what we do say, how we say it and when we say it, makes all the difference between helping and not helping our patients."

–John Apley

"The prime goal of a doctor is to alleviate suffering and not to prolong life. And if your treatment does not alleviate suffering, but only prolongs life, that treatment should be stopped."

–Christiaan Barnard

"Men who occupied the restoration of health in other men, by joint exertion of skills and humanity, are above all the great on the earth. They even partake of divinity, since to preserve and renew is almost as noble as to create."

–Voltaire

"No physician, in so far as he is a physician, considers his own good in what he prescribes, but the good of his patient, for the true physician is also a ruler having the human body as a subject, and is not a mere money-maker."

–Plato

"Don't run after money; money will run after you, if you work sincerely and honestly.

–Anonymous

"Primum non nocere"—First, do no harm."

–Hippocrates

"There are some patients whom we cannot help, there are none whom we cannot harm."

–Arthur L. Bloomfield

"Protecting our ethical heritage is not an abstract, pious counsel of perfection. It is the key to our profession's survival."

–Frederick Lowy

"The critical sense and sceptical attitude of the Hippocratic school laid the foundation of modern medicine on broad lines, and we owe *first*, the emancipation of medicine from the shackles of priestcraft and of caste; *secondly*, the conception of medicine as an art based on accurate observation, and as a science, an integral part of the science of man and of nature; *thirdly*, the high moral ideals, expressed in that most 'memorable of human documents' (Gomprez), the Hippocratic oath; and *fourthly*, the conception and realization of medicine as the profession of a cultivated gentleman."

–William Osler

"It is the bounden duty of the civil society to ensure that the medical professionals are not unnecessarily harassed by the complainants who use the criminal process as a tool for pressurizing the medical professionals and hospitals for extracting uncalled for compensation. It would not be conducive to the efficiency of the medical profession, if a doctor is to administer medicine with a halter around his neck......"

–The Supreme Court of India

"Medicine is a business with a soul. Good medicine can do good business. But good business may not make good medicine."

–Naresh Trehan

"There are some patients whom we cannot help, there are none whom we cannot harm."

–AL Broomfield

"....What is not negotiable is that our profession exists to serve the patient, whose interests come first. None but a saint could follow this principle all the time but so many doctors have followed it so much of the time that the profession has been generally held in high regard."

–Theodore Fox

"Is it not also true that no physician, in so far as he is a physician, considers or enjoins what is for physician's interest, but that all seek the good of their patients? For we have agreed that a physician strictly so called, is a ruler of bodies, and not a maker of money, have we not?"

–Plato

"Some doctors seem to think that MD actually stands for Minor Deity."

–Anonymous

"Many parents are still grateful even if we are unable to save their child... only if we showed concern, care and compassion... and made them perceive that what was humanely possible in the circumstances was done for their baby."

—Meharban Singh

"Ethical decisions are based upon a system of values that serves the best interest of the society in a humane and caring way."

—Anonymous

"...Though shalt behave and act without arrogance and with undistracted mind, humility and constant reflection, thou shalt pray for the welfare of all creatures..."

—Charak Samhita

"Physicians are both morally and legally accountable to the society."

—Anonymous

"Only one rule in medical ethics need concern—that action on your part which best conserves the interests of your patient."

—Martin H. Fischer

"We try never to forget that medicine is for the people. It is not for the profits. The profits follow, and if we have remembered that, they have never failed to appear.

—George Wilhelm Merck

"Remember the first dictum of patient care is "Do No Harm."

—Florence Nightingale

"The right to die is the last and greatest human freedom."

—HL Mencken

"The doctor's aim is to do good, even to our enemies, so much more to our friends, and our profession forbids us to do harm to our kindred, as it is instituted for the benefit and welfare of the human race, and God imposed on physician the oath not to compose mortiferous remedies."

–Rhazes

"The patients will never care how much you know, until they know how much you care."

–Terry Canale

"Medicine is a mission. It is not a profession and it is not a business."

–Mother Teresa

"Physician-assisted suicide and euthanasia have been profound ethical issues confronting doctors since the birth of western medicine, more than 2000 years ago."

–Ezekiel Emanuel

"Only one rule in medical ethics need concern you—that action on your part which best serves the interests of your patient."

–Martin H. Fischer

"Never let your tongue say a slighting word of a colleague."

–William Osler

"Patients may forget your name but they will never forget how you made them feel."

–Maya Angelou

"From the day you begin practice never under any circumstances listen to a tale told to the detriment of a brother practitioner. And when any dispute or trouble does arise, go frankly, ere sunset, and talk the matter over, in which way you may gain a brother and a friend."

–William Osler

"Do not be self-confident about your spiritual progress unless you have reached to the very extinction of all desire."

–Buddha

"Your vision will become clear only when you look into your own heart. Who looks outside, dreams. Who looks inside, awakens."

–Carl Jung Gustav

"Show me a sane man and I will cure him for you."

–Carl Jung Gustav

"It is nice to be a well-informed and skillful physician but it is much nicer to be a good human being. We should strive to master the sublime art of medicine and acquire the divine gift of healing."

–Meharban Singh

"Medicine rests upon four pillars—philosophy, astronomy, alchemy and ethics. The *first* pillar is philosophical knowledge of earth and water; the *second* astronomy, which supplies its full understanding of that which is of fiery and airy nature (celestial or non-earth objects), the *third* is an adequte explanation of the properties of all the four elements—that is to say the whole cosmos—and an introduction into the art of their transformations (from ordinary to extraordinary); and finally, the *fourth* (ethics) shows the physician those virtues which must stay with him up until his death, and it should support and complete the three other pillars."

–Paracelsus

"I am a physician I keep a drug-shop of lies. I give relief and consolation. Can one console and relieve without lying?... Only women and doctors know how necessary and how helpful lies are to men."

–Anatole France

Health, Healing, Faith and Hope

"Health is a state of complete physical, mental and social well being and not merely the absence of disease or infirmity. The enjoyment of highest attainable standard of health is one of the fundamental rights of every human being without distinction of race, religion, political belief, economic or social condition."

−World Health Organization 1946

"The Sanskrit word for health is *swasthya* which means being stabilized in the self. When the mind is free of fear, free of guilt, free of anger and hatred, it has the power to heal the body of any ailment — there is such a huge power in our consciousness."

−Sri Sri Ravi Shankar

"Those who think they have no time for exercise, will sooner or later have to find time for illness."

−Edward Stanley

"Health is like money, we never have a true idea of its value until we lose it."

−Josh Billings

"Time and health are two precious assets that we don't recognize and appreciate until they have been depleted."

−Denis Waitley

"Your body is a temple, but only of you treat it as one."

—Astrid Alauda

"All healing is first healing of the heart."

—Carl Townsend

"Time is the best doctor."

—Ovid

"Healing is not a science but the intuitive art of wooing nature."

—WH Auden

"The physician heals, nature makes well."

—Aristotle

"To keep the body in good health is a duty, for otherwise we shall not be able to trim the lamp of wisdom, and keep our mind strong and clear."

—Buddha

"God heals and doctor takes the fee!"

—Benjamin Franklin

"Your lifestyle, how you live, eat, emote, and think, determines your health. To prevent disease you may have to change how you live."

—Brian Carter

"There are three things which build and maintain civilization throughout the time: pure air, pure water and pure food."

—Zenda Avesta

"It's supposed to be professional secret, but I will tell you anyway. We doctor's do nothing, we only help and encourage the doctor within."

—Albert Scheweitzer

"The best six doctors anywhere—and no one can deny it—are sunshine, water, rest, air, exercise and diet. These six will gladly attend you if only you are willing, your mind they will mend. And charge you not a shilling."

—Wayne Fields

"Turning the face towards God brings healing to the body, the mind and the soul."

—Abdu'ul-Baha

"Body and soul cannot be separated for purposes of treatment, for they are one and indivisible. Sick minds must be healed as well as sick bodies."

—C. Jeff Miller

"To augment the process of healing, the patient must have faith in his doctor and the doctor must have faith in himself and his medicines."

—Meharban Singh

"The physician should not treat the disease but the patient who is suffering from it."

—Maimonides bin Musa

"Laughter is the most healthful exercise; it is one of the greatest helps to digestion with which I am acquainted; and the custom prevalent among our forefathers, of exciting it at table by Jesters and buffoons, was in accordance with sound medical principles."

—Christoph Wilhelm Hufeland

"If we could give every individual the right amount of nourishment and exercise, not too little and not too much, we would have found the safest way to health."

—Hippocrates

"Health is a state of complete harmony of the body, mind and spirit. When one is free from medical disabilities and mental distractions, the gates of the soul open."

—BKS Iyenger

"The doctor may listen and analyze in a more detailed way and use the latest techniques and technologies. But the real physician is a healer, perhaps with a natural talent or gift of healing."

—John Zawacki

"The people who trust their doctor and surrender themselves to his care are more likely to recover than those who approach medicine with distrust, fear and antagonism."

—Anonymous

"In the sick room, ten cents' worth of human understanding equals ten dollars' worth of medical science."

—Martin H. Fischer

"The confidence of the patient in his physician does more for cure of the disease than the physician with all his remedies."

—Henri de Mondevilli

"Vitality and beauty are gifts of nature for those who live according to its laws."

—Leonard da Vinci

"The medical profession has become very used to thinking in terms of doing something to a passive recipient. But patients have to be active participants to augment the process of healing."

—David Felten

"Two things do prolong your life, a quiet heart and a loving wife."

—Indian Proverb

"The physician's highest calling, his only calling, is to make sick people healthy—to heal, as it is termed."

–Samuel Hahnemann

"Our genes can be influenced by every single biological, ecological or behavioral action. We can control about 95% of our genes to improve our biological age."

–Deepak Chopra

"Kindness and a generous spirit go a long way. And a sense of humor, it's like medicine—very healing."

–Max Irons

"Can we afford to ignore the role of emotions, hope, the will to live, the power of human warmth and touch just because they are so difficult to investigate scientifically and our ignorance is so overwhelming?"

–David Felten

"There is nothing that wastes the body like worry does, and one who has any faith in God should be ashamed to worry about anything."

–Mahatma Gandhi

"The greatest wealth is health."

–Virgil

"The art of healing comes from nature and not from the physician. Therefore, the physician must start from nature and with an open mind."

–Paracelsus

"It's not the strongest that survive, neither is it the most intelligent, but those most responsive to change."

–Charles Darwin

"Nothing in life is more wonderful than faith—the one great moving force which we can neither weigh in the balance nor test in the crucible."

–William Osler

"If only people knew the healing power of laughter and joy, many of our fine doctors would be out of business."

–Catherine Ponder

"Confidence and hope do more than the physician."

–Galen

"Prayer indeed is good, but while calling on the gods, a man should himself lend a helping hand."

–Hippocrates

"Our prayers should be for a sound mind in a healthy body."

–Juvenal

"When you are called to see a sick man, be sure you know what the matter is — if you know not, nature can do a great deal better than you can guess."

–Nicholas de Belleville

"Faith and knowledge lean largely upon each other in the practice of medicine."

–Peter Mere Latham

"When you treat a disease, first treat the mind."

–Chen Jen

"Best cure for the body is a quiet mind."

–Napolean Bonaparte

"A wise man should consider that health is the greatest of all human blessings and learn how by his own thoughts he can derive benefit from his illness."

–Hippocrates

"Always make the patient feel that he will be cured (even when you are not convinced of it) for it aids the healing effort of Nature!"

–Hebrew

"The functions of medicine are three fold, to relieve pain, reduce the violence of disease, and to refrain from trying to cure those whom disease has conquered, acknowledging that in such a case medicine is powerless."

–Hippocrates

"Flowers always make people better, happier, and more helfpul. They are sunshine, food and medicine for the soul."

–Luther Burbank

"To keep the body in good health is a duty...... otherwise we shall not be able to keep our mind strong and clear."

–Buddha

"Patients do not put their trust in machines and devices. They put their trust in you."

–Margaret Humburg

"Our power to heal people seems to have diminished as dramatically as our power to cure diseases has increased."

–Bernie Siegel

"All that man needs for health and healing has been provided by God in nature, the challenge of science is to find it."

–Paracelsus

"Restore a man to his health, his purse lies open to thee."

–Robert Burton

"Loving yourself is healing the world."

–Jaymie Gerard

"Day and night, however, thou mayest be engaged, thou shalt endeavor for the relief of patients with all thy heart and soul. Thou shalt not desert or injure thy patient even for the sake of thy life or thy living. Thy behavior must be in consideration of time and place and heedful of past experience. Thou shalt act always with a view to the acquisition of knowledge...... There is no limit at all to the science of life, medicine. So thou should apply thyself to it with diligence."

—Charaka

"If you trust Google more than your doctor then may be its time to find another doctor."

—Cristina Cordova

"So many come to the sickroom thinking of themselves as men of science fighting disease and not as healers with a little knowledge of helping nature to get a sick man well."

—Auckland Geddes

"Empolyment is nature's physician and is essential to human happiness."

—Galen

"Laughter is the best medicine but if you laugh for no reason, you need medicine."

—Author Unknown

"We have not lost faith, but we have transferred it from God to the medical profession."

—George Bernard Shaw

"We ought to know our body better than a doctor, for we live in it all the time. We must perceive what invigorates or violates it in response to environment, food, life style, moods and thoughts—that awareness is indeed the best health promotive mantra."

—Meharban Singh

"Health is love, joy, enthusiasm, achievement, expression and service. Not mere absence of disease; it is a dynamic expression of life."

—Sri Sri Ravi Shankar

"The people go and beseech the gods for health and do not know, that they themselves have the power over it."

—Democrat

"Without faith a man can do nothing; with it all things are possible."

—William Osler

"If you do not believe in yourself how can you expect other people to do so? If you have not an abiding faith in the profession you cannot be happy in it."

—William Osler

"To the sick, while there is life, there is hope."

—Cicero

"Thinking of disease constantly will intensify it. Feel always 'I am healthy in body and mind'."

—Swami Sivananda

"He who has health, has hope; and he who has hope, has everything."

—Thomas Fuller

"Hope is the poor man's bread."

—Thales

"Drugs are not always necessary, but belief in recovery always is."

—Norman Cousins

"Feed a cold and starve a fever."

—Indian Proverb

"Love, hope, peace and joy have physiological consequences, just as depression and despair do."

—Bernie Siegel

"Hope and love cures people whom medicine and surgery can't. Nobody's disease is hopeless, but many people are."

—Karl Meninger

"Never go to a doctor, whose office plants have died."

—Erma Bombeck

"If body is feeble, the mind will not be strong."

—Thomas Jefferson

"Everyone has a doctor in him or her, we just have to help it in its work. The natural healing force within each one of us is the greatest force in getting well. Our food should be our medicine. But to eat when you are sick, is to feed your sickness."

—Hippocrates

"There are 100 trillion plus beneficial microorganisms in our microbiome that resides in our mouth, gastrointestinal system and skin. When there is imbalance in our microbiome (due to faulty lifestyle, unhealthy diet, unnecessary drugs), it leads to inflammation in various body organs which is a trigger for a large number of diseases."

—Deepak Chopra

"Our Creator has given us five senses to help us survive threats from the external world, and a sixth sense, our healing system, to help us survive internal threats. There is much we can do, as individuals, to activate or impede this healing system."

—Bernie Siegel

"Our healing capabilities are mobilized by love, faith, living in the moment, forgiveness and hope."

–Bernie Siegel

"Anything that offers hope has the potential to heal, including thoughts, suggestions, symbols and placebos."

–Anonymous

"Medicine is a synonym for healing. It is healing of the afflictions of air, bile and phlegm of the body. It is the healing of the afflictions of desire, hatred and ignorance of the mind."

–Zurkharpa Lodro Gyaltshen

"Our sorrows and wounds are healed only when we touch them with compassion."

–Buddha

"God healeth and physician hath the thanks."

–English Proverb

"What is the wisest among the human matters? The art of healing!"

–Pythogoras

"Arouse the energy and wisdom within you for healing. And harness the sources, essence and forces of power around; the sun, moon, space, water, a river, the ocean, air, fire, trees, flowers, people, animals, light, sound, smell, taste and any aspect of energy that one finds inspiring and healing."

–Buddhist Doctrine

"If we could give every individual the right amount of nourishment and exercise, not too little and not too much, we would have found the safest way to health."

–Hippocrates

"Our minds possess the power of healing pain and creating joy. If we use that power along with proper living, a positive attitude, and meditation, we can heal not only our mental and emotional afflictions, but even physical problems."

—Buddhist Doctrine

"When you look at others with a smiling, kind and caring eyes, the act of looking becomes a prayer, a meditation and a way of healing, when you see the outside world with calmness and clarity, your inner self reflects positive energy like a mirror."

—Anonymous

"Medicine to produce health must examine disease and music to create harmony, must investigate discord."

—Plutarch

"To promote the healing response, you must get past all the grosser levels of the body—cells, tissues, organs and systems—and arrive at a junction between mind and matter, the point where consciousness actually starts to have an effect."

—Deepak Chopra

"And when you are in great pain, ask the 'healing light' to help you. Imagine from your fingers emanate rays of light of every color and train these rays on the painful area. You will soon feel a gradual release from pain."

—Omraam Mikhael Aivanhov

"Before healing others, heal yourself."

—Lao Tzu

"Health is not simply absence of sickness."

—Hannah Green

"Nothing is more fatal to health than an over care of it."

—Benjamin Franklin

"Faith and prayer are vitamins of the soul; man cannot live in health without them."

–Mahalia Jackson

"Your love can be harnessed to become a great and wonderful healing force."

–Richard Gordon

"Have you ever wondered why people immediately and automatically put their hands on whatever part of their body is injured? It seems this action is universal and built into our neural hardware because it promotes the process of healing."

–Richard Gordon

"Physical illness is not only one of the most important keys to a healthy body, it is the basis for dynamic and creative intellectual activity."

–John F. Kennedy

"Life force energy has been acknowledged, appreciated and utilized by numerous cultures around the world for thousand of years. The Chinese call it 'chi' and the Japanese call it 'ki'. The Indian yogis have called the energy 'prana' and have used their understanding to achieve higher levels of consciousness through various practices of yoga, pranayama, meditation and visualization to promote healing. The Hawaiian Kahunas referred to it as 'mana' and used it for hands-on healing, distant healing and for prayer."

–Anonymous

"Hope is the greatest healer — anything that offers hope has the potential to heal whether it is a suggestion, thought, symbol or placebo."

–Bernie Siegel

"Natural forces within us are the true healers of disease."

–Hippocrates

"He who has health has hope; and to he who has hope has everything."

–Arab Proverb

"A good laugh and long sleep are the best cures in the doctor's book."

–Irish Proverb

"Faith and knowledge lean largely upon each other in the practice of medicine."

–Peter Mere Latham

"Refuse to be ill. Never tell people you are ill, never own it to yourself. Illness is one of those things which a man should resist on principle at the outset."

–Bulwer-Lytton

"I dressed him, and God healed him."

–Ambroise Pare

"To the sick, while there is life, there is hope."

–Cicero

"The physician cures, nature makes well."

–Aristotle

"Patience is the art of hoping."

–Marquis de Vauvenargues

"Prayer is the voice of faith."

–Horne

"Love is the best medicine and there is more than enough to go around once you open your heart."

–Julie Marie

"Hope, faith, love and compassion have great healing powers."

—*Bernie Siegel*

"There is no doubt that there is a connection between what we ingest, what we wear, what we feel, and the way our immune system responds."

—*Richard Mucci*

"Pray as if everything depended on God, and work as if everything depended upon man."

—*FC Spellman*

"Of all the healers, O Spitama Zarathustra namely those who heal with knife, with herbs, and with sacred incantations, the last one is the most potent as he heals from the very source of diseases."

—*Ardihesht Yasht*

"Look upon every man, woman and everyone as God. You cannot help anyone, you can only serve, serve the children of the Lord Himself, if you have the privilege."

—*Swami Vivekananda*

"The doctor's character can influence the patients' recovery more than any medicine."

—*Paracelsus*

"Each illness has a musical solution. The shorter and more complete the solution — the greater the musical talent of the physician. Sickness demands manifold solutions. The selection of the most appropriate solution determines the talent of the physician."

—*Novalis*

"Then comes the question, how do drugs, hygiene and magnetism heal? It may be affirmed that they do not heal, but only relieve suffering temporarily, exchanging one disease for another."

—Mary Baker Eddy

"Take the torch of your mind to the areas you feel pain; light the area with the light of your graceful awareness and then visualize the divine grace healing that pain and affliction."

—Shuddaanandaa Brahmachari

"In the deserts of the heart, let the healing fountain start."

—WH Auden

"It is part of the cure to wish to be cured."

—Seneca

"There is a light in this world, a healing spirit more powerful than any darkness we may encounter. We sometime lose sight of this force when there is suffering, and too much pain. Then suddenly, the spirit will emerge through the lives of ordinary people who hear a call and answer in extraordinary ways."

—Mother Teresa

"Heal others without revealing yourself as a healer. Your capacity to heal will be enhanced."

—Swami Veda Bharti

"Disease is a lack of health. Health is not a lack of disease."

—Author Unknown

"The church says, the body is a sin. Science says, the body is a machine. Advertising says, the body is a business. The body says, I am a fiesta."

—Eduardo Galeano

"When health is absent, wisdom cannot reveal itself, art cannot manifest, strength cannot fight, wealth becomes useless and intelligence cannot be applied."

–Herophilus

"The four pillars of good health are sound genetic constitution, safe environment, wholesome food and healthy life style."

–Meharban Singh

"The doctor has been taught to be interested in disease. What the public should be taught that the health is the cure for disease."

–Ashley Montagu

"Treatment originates outside you, healing comes from within."

–Andrew Weil

"Hospitals should be arranged in such a way as to make being sick an interesting experience. One learns a great deal sometimes from being sick."

–Alan W. Watts

"Healing is a matter of time, but it is sometimes also a matter of opportunity."

–Hippocrates

"Health can be defined negatively, as the absence of illness, functionally as the ability to cope with everyday activities, or positively as fitness and wellbeing. It has also been noted in the modern world that health has a moral and spiritual dimension."

–Mildred Baxter

"The human body contains blood, phlegm, yellow bile and black bile. These are the things that make up its constitution and cause its pain and health. Health is primarily that state in which these consituents are present in the correct proportion to each other, both in strength and quantity, and are well mixed."

–*Hippocrates*

"Wisdom is to the soul, what health is to the body."

–*La Rouchefoucauld*

"Simply put, music can heal people."

–*Harry Reid*

"Health is the proper relationship between microcosm, which is man, and the macrocosm, which is the universe. Disease is a disruption of this relationship."

–*Yeshe Donden*

"I believe that you can, by taking some simple and inexpensive measures, extend your life and your years of wellbeing. My most important recommendation is that you take vitamins every day in optimum amounts, to supplement the vitamins you receive in your food."

–*Linus Pauling*

"A careful physician, before he attempts to administer a remedy to his patient must investigate not only the malady of the man he wishes to cure, but also his habits when in health and his physical constitution."

–*Cicero*

"Every human being is the author of his own health or disease."

–*Sivananda*

"Pain is inevitable. Suffering is optional."

–*M. Kathleen Casey*

"By cleansing your body on a regular basis and eliminating as many toxins as possible from your environment, your body can begin to heal itself, prevent disease, and become stronger and more resilient than you ever dreamed possible!"

–Edward F. Group

"Rest, as soon as there is pain, is a great restorative of all disturbances of the body."

–Hippocrates

"There is no curing a sick man who believes himself in health."

–Henri Amiel

"The more serious the illness, the more important it is for you to fight back mobilizing all your resources—physical, intellectual, emotional and spiritual."

–Norman Cousins

"The era of survival of the fittest is over and replaced by the mantra of survival of the wisest. Your attitude of gratitude, positive thinking, relaxation and medication can reduce inflammation, improve immunity and biological age."

–Deepak Chopra

"It is often thought that medicine is the curative process. It is no such thing; nature alone cures. And what nursing has to do is, to put the patient in the best condition for nature to act upon him."

–Florence Nightingale

"If we could give every individual the right amount of nourishment and exercise, not too little and not too much, we would have found the safest way to health."

–Hippocrates

"Natural forces within us are the true healers of disease."

–Hippocrates

"Prayer indeed is good, but while calling on gods, a man should himself lend a hand."

–Hippocrates

"Cure sometimes, treat often, comfort always."

–Hippocrates

"In the deserts of the heart, let the healing fountain start."

–WH Auden

"The world does not need a new medicine. It needs doctors who know how to pray and obey God in their own lives. In such hands, medicine with all its modern resources, will bring forth fruits in abundance."

–Paul Tournier

History of Medicine

A Short History of Medicine

2000 BC "Here, eat this root."

1000 BC "That root is heathen, say this prayer."

1850 AD "That prayer is no good, drink this potion."

1940 AD "That potion is snake oil, swallow this pill."

1985 AD "That pill is ineffective, take this antibiotic."

2000 AD "That antibiotic is spurious. Here, eat this root."

—Author Unknown

"The history of medicine is not the testament of idealistic seekers after health and life...... The history of medicine is largely the substitution of ignorance by fallacies..."

—Richard Gordon

"Medical writings of the Middle Ages set great store by astrology. What went on in each part of the body was determined by the influence of the planets and signs of Zodiac. The sun ruled the right hand side of the body, the moon the left, venus the neck and abdomen, and so on."

—Paracelsus

Holistic Medicine

"Health depends on a state of equilibrium among various factors that govern the operation of the body and the mind; the equilibrium in turn is reached only when man lives in harmony with his external environment."

—Hippocrates

"It is more important to know what sort of person has a disease than what sort of disease a person has."

—Hippocrates

"Doctors who persist in thinking that they can cure the disease without caring for the person may be excellent technicians but they are incomplete doctors."

—Anonymous

"The cure of many diseases remains unknown to the physicians of Hellos (Greece) because they do not study the whole person."

—Socrates

"The patients should not be viewed as systems, organs, tissues, cells and DNA. They must be viewed in totality (body, mind, heart and soul) and that too not in isolation but in context with the dynamics of ecology, family, friends and society."

—Meharban Singh

"Medicine is about sick people, not diseases."

—William Osler

"No two patients are alike though they may have the same disease. Never ignore the uniqueness and individuality of every patient and his ecology. Understand and unfold its mysteries to ensure comprehensive care and global healing rather than mere cure........"

–Meharban Singh

"Mind, Spirit and Body hold life in balance with the three doshas like a pot on three supports."

–Charaka

"The poets did well to conjoin music and medicine in Apollo, because the philosophy of medicine is but to tune this curious harp of man's body and to reduce it to harmony."

–Francis Bacon

"For many people, managing pain involves using prescription medicine in combination with complementary techniques like physical therapy, acupuncture, yoga and massage. I appreciate this because I truly believe medical care should address the person as a whole—their body, mind and spirit."

–Naomi Judd

"When one has fallen ill, one must change one's way of life. It is clear that the life one has been living is bad altogether, or in part, or in some respect..."

–Hippocrates

"Medicine alone takes as its province the whole man.... It is concerned with man in all the complexity of his body and mind from his conception to his last breath; and its concerns extend increasingly beyond his sicknesses, to the conditions which make it possible for him to lead a healthy and a happy life."

–Russell Brain

"For the most part, western medicine doctors are not healers, preventers, listeners, or educators. But they're damn good at saving a life and the other aspects kick the beam. It's about time we brought some balance back to the scale."

–Claire Todae

"Doctors who treat the symptom tend to give a prescription; doctors who treat the patient are more likely to offer guidance."

–John Apley

"Once a disease has entered the body, all parts which are healthy must fight it, not one alone, but all. Because a disease might mean their common death. Nature knows this; and nature attacks the disease with whatever help she can muster."

–Paracelsus

"When you treat a disease, first treat the mind."

–Chen Jen

"It is with disease of the mind, as with those of the body; we are half-dead before we understand our disorder, and half cured when we do."

–Colton C. Charles

"A bodily disease which we look upon as whole and entire within itself, may, after all, be but a symptom of some ailment in the spiritual part."

–Nathaniel Hawthorne

"Variability is the law of life, and as no two faces are the same, so no two bodies are alike, and no two individuals react alike and behave alike under the abnormal conditions which we know as disease."

–William Osler

"Here's good advice for practice: Go into partnership with nature; she does more than half the work and asks none of the fee."

–*Martin H. Fischer*

"The essence of practice of medicine is that it is an intensely personal matter. The treatment of a disease may be entirely impersonal; the care of the patient must be completely personal."

–*Francis W. Peabody*

"The majority of the diseases which the human family have been and still are suffering under, they got created by ignorance of their own organic health, and work perseveringly to tear themselves to pieces, and when broken down and debilitated in body and mind, send for the doctor and drug themselves to death."

–*Ellen White*

"The modern medicine is depersonalized science in the service of prolonging life rather than diminishing human suffering."

–*Elisabeth Kübler-Ross*

"...What happens then is like what happens when we separate a jigsaw puzzle into its five hundred pieces. The over-all picture disappears. This is the state of modern medicine. It has lost the sense of the unity of man. Such is the price it has paid for its scientific progress. It has sacrificed art to science."

–*Paul Tournier*

"The practice of medicine will be very much as you make it—to one a worry, a care, a perpetual annoyance; to another, a daily job and a life of as much happiness and usefulness as can well fall to the lot of man, because it is a life of self-sacrifice and of countless opportunities to comfort and help the weak-hearted, and to raise up those that fall."

−William Osler

"Life is short, science is long, opportunity is elusive, experiment is dangerous, and judgement is difficult. It is not enough for the physician to do what is necessary, but the patient and attendants must do their part as well, and circumstances must be favorable."

−Hippocrates

"The doctor of the future will give no medicine but will interest his patients in the care of the human frame, in diet and in the cause and prevention of disease."

−Thomas Edison

"The more I work with the body, keeping my assumptions in a temporary state of reservation, the more I appreciate and sympathize with a given 'disease'... The body no longer appears as a sick or irrational demon, but as a process with its own inner logic and wisdom."

−Arnold Mindell

"...Pituitary gland has a connection to the hypothalamus gland, which is the seat of consciousness, our mind. Thousands of years ago, people had stated that focus of pituitary gland can affect the whole nervous system in a very positive way. Consciousness works through glands and cleans and brings energy into the immune system, strengthens it and keeps one healthy or *swasthya* which means stabilized in one's self. Health means that mind is centered, focused, free of disturbances and solid."

−Sri Sri Ravi Shankar

"Even though everyone has two eyes, two ears, a nose and a mouth, there are no two faces exactly alike. Though the

DNA is a common denominator to us all, to billions of us, it still manages to create each single human being as a unique individual."

—Tom Laughlin

"Living in peace, free from emotional afflictions, and loosening our grip on "self" is the ultimate medicine both for mental and physical health."

—Tibetan Doctrine

"Modern medicine is still dominated by the notion that disease is caused by adverse external agents. But Ayurveda believes that host is all-important and disease cannot take hold unless host accepts it."

—Ayurvedic Doctrine

"All the Ayurvedic healing techniques operate on the premise that one treats the patient first, the disease second."

—Deepak Chopra

"A physician is obligated to consider a patient more than a diseased organ, more even than the whole man—he must view the man in his world."

—Harvey Cushing

"Disharmony between body and mind is the root cause of sickness."

—Buddha

"Disease happens when things get out of balance. For example, there is nothing wrong with cells dividing and multiplying in the body but when this process continues in disregard of the total organism, cells continue to proliferate and we have the disease."

—Eckhart Tolle

"For many people, managing pain involves using prescription medicines in combination with complementary techniques like physical therapy, acupuncture, yoga and massage. I appreciate this because I truly believe medical care should address the person as a whole—their body, mind and spirit."

—Naoi Judel

Laboratory Investigations

"The physician should have faith in his clinical acumen and should treat the patient and not his laboratory reports......"

–John Apley

"Use the laboratory as your slave, not the savior. Because slavish submission to the laboratory reports may lead to the atrophy of the clinical judgement."

–Meharban Singh

"Whoever thought up the word "mammogram"? Everytime I hear it, I think I'm supposed to put my breast in an envelope and send it to someone."

–Jan King

15

Mind, Thoughts and Habits

"If we'll open our minds to study how emotions influence our health, then may be we'll eventually open our minds towards the spiritual dimensions of health."

—John Zawacki

"Every day doctors have to deal with people who are worn out and unable to stand up to the life they lead. They generally assert that it is impossible to alter the way they live, and sincerely believe that their overwork is the product of circumstance, whereas it is bound up with their own intimate problems. It is ambition, fear of the future, love of money, jealousy, or social injustice that makes men strive and overwork, invent all sorts of unnecessary tasks, keep late hours, take too little sleep, take insufficient holidays, or use their holidays badly. Their minds are overtense, so that at night they cannot sleep and by day they doubly fatigue themselves at their work."

—Paul Tournier

"The child is the barometer of family's emotional climate. Behavioral and psychological problems in children are a reflection of inter-parental marital conflicts......"

—John Apley

"We cannot prevent the birds of sadness from flying over our heads but we must not let them build a nest in our hair."

—Chinese Proverb

"Habit is a cable, we weave a thread of it every day, and at last we cannot break it."

–Horace Mann

"Fortunately psychoanalysis is not the only way to resolve inner conflicts. Life itself remains a very effective therapist."

–Karen Horney

"Every human being is the author of his own health or disease."

–Buddha

"Analysis is the way of mind, hugging is the way of heart. The mind is the cause of all diseases and the heart is the source of all healing."

–Osho

"Mild behavioral and emotional disturbances are like the common cold, everyone suffers or sniffs at times, though some people won't blow their noses in public."

–John Apley

"Do not diagnose a psychosomatic or emotional disorder only because there is no evidence of organic disease. You should also have positive evidences of an emotional disturbance."

–John Apley

"Habits are first cobwebs, then cables."

–Spanish Proverb

"Live the each present moment completely, and the future will take care of itself. Fully enjoy the wonder and beauty of each instant."

–Parmahansa Yogananda

"It seems that the second half of a man's life is made up of nothing but the habits he has accumulated during the first half."

—Feodor Dostoevski

"We are what we think. All that we are arises with our thoughts. With our thoughts, we make our world."

—Buddha

"It is not enough to have a good mind, the main thing is to use it well."

—Rene Descartes

"A sad soul can kill you quicker than a germ."

—John Steinbeck

"That's the most interesting thing of all. The balance depends on the man's frame of mind! Understand? Which means that if he's cheerful and firm in spirit, there will be more sodium in the barrier, and no sickness, none whatsoever, will bring him to his death. But as soon as he loses heart, the potassium gains the upper hand and he might as well order himself a coffin... The physiology of optimism..."

—Alexander Zolzhenitsyn

"The beginning of habit is like an invisible thread, but everytime we repeat the act, we strengthen the strand, add to it another filament, until it becomes a great cable and binds us irrevocably, both in thought and action."

—Orison Swett Marden

"We first make our habits and then our habits make us."

—John Dryden

"I went to medical school because I wanted to ask big questions. Do we have a soul? Does God exist? What happens after death"?

—Deepak Chopra

"A person's mood is like a symphony, and serotonin is like conductor's baton."

–James Stockard

"Your lifestyle—how you live, eat, emote and think determines your health. To prevent disease, you may have to change how you live ."

–Brian Carter

"When you are feeling stressed and about to break—just remember STRESSED is simply DESSERTS spelled backwards—it's a piece of cake and so just enjoy."

–Anonymous

"Anger, anxiety, depression, fear and many other feelings are unhealthy only if they remain buried inside, unexpressed and not dealt with."

–Candace Pert

"Our cells are constantly eavesdropping on our thoughts and are being changed by them. A bout of depression can wreak havoc with the immune system, falling in love can boost it. Joy and fulfillment keep us healthy and extend life."

–Deepak Chopra

"Above all, don't lose your desire to walk, everyday I walk myself into a state of well-being and walk away from illness. I have walked myself into my best thoughts. Thus, if one keeps on walking, everything will be all right."

–Kierkegourd

"You become what you think about."

–Earl Nightingale

"The mind is in all cells of the body. Every cell in our body is having conversation with each other all the time even during sleep. The healthy mind is indeed the key to health and wellbeing."

–Deepak Chopra

"Most people find it much easier to hold on to negative thoughts than the positive ones. On an average, a person can hold a positive thought for only 4–7 seconds, whereas we worry for hours, days or even years about something that hasn't yet happened!"

–Anonymous

"My life has been filled with the most dreadful misfortune most of which never happened."

–Michel de Montaigne

"The thoughts that come often unsought, and, as it were, drop into the mind, are commonly the most valuable of any we have."

–John Locke

"…When we learn to laugh at ourselves and our problems, we heal. When we learn to enjoy ourselves and refrain from seeing problems as negative, we become more positive about everything. Positive thinking is a wonderful habit to develop, for it heals us and makes us happy in our lives…"

–Dodrupchen

"If you can solve your problem, then what is the need of worrying? If you cannot solve it, then what is the use of worrying?"

–Shantideva

"The mind can be likened to an iceberg. The part above the surface of water is the conscious mental activity. The submerged mass, comprising 90%, is the unconscious, unseen but powerful. Most of us use less than 5% of our brainpower!"

–David Swindley

"The unconscious mind contains all your memories, dreams and fantasies and is the part of the mind, which generates new, creative ideas, often without involving the conscious mind at all."

−Carl Jung Gustav

"Individuals create their own unique life styles and are, therefore, responsible for their own personality and behavior. They are creative actors rather than passive reactors."

−Alfred Adler

"You take control of your life by taking control of your thoughts. Transform your thinking, and you transform your life."

−Rex Johnson

"Habit, if not resisted, soon becomes a necessity."

−St. Augustine

"Health is not a condition of matter, but of mind; nor can the material senses bear reliable testimony on the subject of health."

−Mary Baker Eddy

"The kingdom of heaven is not a place but a state of mind."

−J. Burroughs

"The mind in its own place and in itself can make a heaven of hell, a hell of heaven."

−Milton

"Nothing is so fatal to the progress of the human mind as to suppose that our views of science are ultimate, that there are no mysteries in nature, that our triumphs are complete, and that there are no new worlds to conquer."

−Humphry Davy

"The part can never be well, unless the whole is well."
—Plato

"If the essential core of the person is denied or suppressed, he gets sick, sometimes in obvious ways, sometimes in subtle ways, sometimes immediately, sometimes later."
—Abraham Maslow

"Worry, not the work, kills a man."
—Maltese Proverb

"Worry is stomach's worst poison."
—Alfred Nobel

"The mind is a great healer."
—Hippocrates

"A merry heart doeth good like medicine."
—English Proverb

"He who sings frighten away his ills."
—Cervantes

"For each bad emotion, our system generates injurious chemical compounds while agreeable and happy emotions are associated with production of life-sustaining nutritious chemicals."
—Elmer C. Gates

"When the breath wanders, the mind is also unsteady. But when the breath is calmed, the mind too becomes still and the yogi achieves a long life."
—Svatmarama

"If you are depressed you are living in the past. If you are anxious, you are living in the future. If you are at peace, you are living in the present."
—Lao Tzu

16

Miracles and Mysticism

"Whether they admit it as much or denied it, they all without exception in the depths of their hearts believed that there was a doctor, or a herbalist, or some old witch of a woman somewhere, whom you only had to find and get that medicine... to be saved.... It just wasn't possible that their lives were already doomed. However, much we laugh at miracles when we are strong, healthy and prosperous, if life becomes so hedged and cramped that only a miracle can save us, then we clutch at this unique, exceptional miracle and – believe in it!"

–Alexander Solzhenitsyn

"Formerly, when religion was strong and science weak, men mistook magic for medicine; now, when science is strong and religion weak, men mistake medicine for magic."

–Thomas Szasz

"We rationalize, we dissimilate, we pretend that modern medicine is a rational science, all facts, no nonsense, and just what it seems. But we have only to tap its glossy veneer for it to split wide open, and reveal to us its roots and foundations, its old dark heart of metaphysics, mysticism, magic and myth."

–Oliver Sacks

"There are two ways to live your life. One is though nothing is a miracle. The other is as though everything is a miracle."

–Albert Einstein

17

Miscellaneous Concerns and Issues

"Health is a state of complete physical, mental, social and spiritual wellbeing, and not merely the absence of disease or infirmity."

—World Health Organization 1948

"To understand any living thing, you must peep within and feel the beating of its heart."

—W. Macneile Dixon

"It is only with the heart that one can see rightly. What is essential is invisible to the eye."

—Antoine de Saint-Exupéry

"The best doctors anywhere and no one can deny it, are sunshine, water, rest, air, exercise and diet."

—Wayne Fields

"He who laughs, lasts."

—Victor Borge

"Always laugh when you can, it is a cheap medicine."

—George Gordon Byron

"God will only mend a broken heart when He is given all the pieces."

—Anonymous

"The three, i.e. body, mind and soul are like a tripod, the world stands by their combination, in them everything abides."

—Charaka Samhita

"Tears are the safety valve of the heart when too much pressure is laid on it."

—Albert Smith

"Nothing is more damaging to health than over care of it."

—Benjamin Franklin

"In spite of everything, I still believe people are really good at heart."

—Anne Frank

"Pain is God's greatest gift to mankind."

—Paul Brand

"Seeds of past *karma* cannot germinate if they are roasted in the fire of divine wisdom."

—Parmahansa Yogananda

"Learn to get in touch with silence within yourself and know that everything in this life has a purpose. There are no mistakes, no coincidences. All events are blessings given to us to learn from."

—Elisabeth Kübler-Ross

"To ensure good health, eat lightly, breathe deeply, live moderately, cultivate cheerfulness, and maintain an interest in life."

—William Londen

"The Divine Alchemist can miraculously change a sorrowing heart of lead into a golden mellowness that sings praises through tears."

—SL McMillen

"One should strive to maintain good health by taking a balanced diet and exercising regularly."

—Atharva Veda

"Do not dwell in the past, do not dream of the future, concentrate the mind on the present moment."

—Buddha

"To live long, live slowly."

−Cicero

"Let me tell you the secret that has let me to my goal. My strength lies solely in my tenacity."

−Louis Pasteur

"Science is the father of knowledge, but opinion breeds ignorance."

−Hippocrates

"Great thoughts come from the heart."

−Marquis de Vauvenargues

"Joy is a net of love by which you can catch souls… A joyful heart is the inevitable result of a heart burning with love."

−Mother Teresa

"A speaker who does not strike oil in ten minutes should stop boring."

−Louis Nizer

"Without love and kindness life is cold, selfish and uninteresting and leads to distaste for everything. With kindness, the difficult becomes easy, the obscure becomes clear; life assumes a charm and its miseries are softened. If we knew the power of kindness, we should transform the world into a paradise."

−Charles Wagner

"The effect of one good-hearted person is incalculable."

−Oscar Arias

"Nurses are the heart of health care."

−Donn Wilk Caudill

"A doctor is often more to be feared than the disease."

−French Proverb

"Heaven defend me from the busy doctor."

—*Welsh Proverb*

"Choose a job you love and you will never have to work a day in your life."

—*Confucius*

"The man is as old as his arteries."

—*Thomas Sydenham*

"Continuing to fill a pail after it is full, the water will be wasted. Continuing to grind an axe after it is sharp, will wear it away. Excess of condiments deadens the taste. He who practices moderation is lasting and enduring. Too much is always a curse, most of all in wealth."

—*Lao Tzu*

"As for me, all I know is that I know nothing."

—*Socrates*

"I have found the paradox that if I love until it hurts, then there is no hurt, but only more love."

—*Mother Teresa*

"We cannot do great things. We can only do small things with great love."

—*Mother Teresa*

"Disease comes on horseback, but goes away on foot."

—*Popular Proverb*

"Nothing is impossible to the willing heart."

—*Thomas Heywood*

"I attribute my success to this—I never gave or took any excuse."

—*Florence Nightingale*

"Our job as nurses is to cushion the sorrow and celebrate the joy, everyday, while we are "just doing our job."

–Christine Belle

"Let us inquire then regarding what is admitted to be medicine; namely that which was invented for the sake of the sick, which possesses a name and practitioners."

–Hippocrates

"It is health that is the real wealth and not pieces of gold and silver."

–Mahatma Gandhi

"Its not the years in your life that count, its life in your years."

–Abraham Lincoln

"Whosoever saves the life of one person, it would be as if he saved the life of all humankind."

–Quran

"Health is the greatest gift, contentment the greatest wealth, faithfulness the best relationship."

–Buddha

"People pay the doctor for his trouble, for his kindness they still remain in his debt."

–Seneca

"Health is not valued until sickness comes."

–Thomas Fuller

"Children are completely egoistic, they feel their needs intensely and strive ruthlessly to satisfy them."

–Sigmund Freud

"From a relatively weak, traditional profession of minor economic significance, medicine has become a sprawling system of hospitals, clinics, health plans, insurance companies, and myriad other organizations employing a vast labor force."

–Paul Starr

"Apollo was held the God of physick, and sender of diseases. Both were originally in the same trade, and still continue."

–Jonathan Swift

"My 'medicine' was the thing that gained me entrance to these secret gardens of the self. It lay there, another world, in the self. I was permitted by my medical badge to follow the poor, defeated body into these gulfs and grottos."

–William Carlos Williams

"Health is better than wealth."

–Popular Saying

"Eat right, exercise regularly, die anyway."

–Author Unknown

"The doctor dresses the wound and God heals it."

–Popular Saying

"An imaginary ailment is worse than a disease."

–Yiddish Proverb

"If your dog is fat, you are not getting enough exercise."

–Author unknown

"Imbalance between microbiome and human cells leads to inflammation, which is the basis for all diseases, may it be infections, autoimmune disorders, diabetes mellitus, heart disease, and several types of cancers."

–Deepak Chopra

"Medicine not merely denotes a kind of knowledge, but it comprehends the various applications of that knowledge to the alleviation of the sufferings, the repair of the injuries, and the conservation of health, of living beings."

–Thomas Henry Huxley

"The secret of health both for the body and mind is not to mourn for the past, not to worry about future but to live the present moment wisely and earnestly."

—Buddha

"The best way to find yourself is to lose yourself in the service of others."

—Mahatma Gandhi

"It is apparently difficult for doctors to understand hypertension as a quantitative, not qualitative disease because it is a departure from the ordinary process of binary thought to which they are brought up. It is normal or abnormal, physiological or pathological, health or disease, good or bad? Quantity is not an idea that is as yet allowed to intrude. Medicine in its present state can count up to two but not beyond."

—George White Pickering

"Men are not going to embrace eugenics. They are going to embrace the first trim-figured girl with limpid eyes and flashing teeth who comes along, in spite of the fact that her germ plasm is probably reeking with hypertension, cancer, hemophilia, color blindness, hay fever, epilepsy, and amyotrophic lateral sclerosis."

—Logan Clendening

"The only way to keep your health is to eat what you don't want, drink what you don't like, and do what you'd rather not."

—Mark Twain

"Your genome is the mirror of your *karma* and *sanskars*."

—Meharban Singh

"In science, the credit goes to the man who convinces the world, not to the man to whom the idea first occurs."

—William Osler

"Look wise, say nothing, and grunt. Speech was given to conceal thought."

—William Osler

"Live neither in the past nor in the future, but let each day's work absorb your entire energies, and satisfy your wildest ambitions."

—William Osler

"The chief worries of life arise from the foolish habit of looking before and after."

—William Osler

"Laughter is a tranquilizer with no side effects."

—Arnold H. Glasow

"Three rules: I do not eat too much, I do not worry too much; and, if I do my best, I believe that what happens, happens for the best."

—Henry Ford

"The trained nurse has become one of the great blessings of humanity, taking a place beside the physician and priest."

—William Osler

"To be idle is a short road to death and to be diligent is a way of life; foolish people are idle, wise people are diligent."

—Buddha

"It is better to be silent and be thought a fool, than to speak and remove all doubt."

—Abraham Lincoln

"Misdirected life force is the activity in disease process. Disease has no energy save what it borrows from the life of the organism. It is by adjusting the life force that healing must be brought about, and it is the sun as transformer and

distributor of primal spiritual energy that must be utilized in this process, for life and the sun are so intimately connected."
—Kabbalah

"He who avoids extremes,
  In feeding and fasting,
  In sleep and walking,
  And in work and play,
  He winnith yoga, balance, peace and joy."
—Bhagavad Gita

"Medicine heals diseases of the body, wisdom frees the soul from passions."
—Democritus

"When you are young, you use your health to chase your wealth. When you are old, you use your wealth to buy back your health."
—Indian Saying

"I think one's feelings waste themselves in words, they ought all to be distilled into actions which bring results."
—Florence Nightingale

"To 'feel fit a fiddle', you must tone down your middle."
—Author Unknown

"Disease is the retribution of outraged nature."
—Hosea Ballou

"Happiness? That's nothing more than good health and a poor memory."
—Albert Schweitzer

"The prerequisite for today's medical policy is naturally the currently predominant system of medicine. The sick are the source of income, therefore, it is necessary for sick people to be there, yes, it proves advantageous if one makes the people artificially sick."

—*Author Unknown*

"Modern medicine is a negation of health. It isn't organized to serve human health, but only itself, as an institution. It makes more people sick than it heals."

—*Ivan Illich*

"We have not lost faith, but we have transferred it from God to the medical profession."

—*George Bernard Shaw*

"Live fast and die young, live slow and die old."

—*Popular Saying*

"The more you know, the less you understand."

—*Lao Tzu*

"Live as if you were to die tomorrow. Learn as if you were to live forever."

—*Mahatma Gandhi*

"The medical establishments have become the major threat to health."

—*Ivan Illich*

"According to Charaka, the nurses should be of good behavior, distinguished for purity, possessed of cleverness and skills, imbued with kindness, skilled in every service a patient may require, competent to cook food, skilled in bathing or sponging the patient, rubbing and massaging the limbs, lifting and assisting him to walk, well skilled in making and cleansing of beds, readying the patient and skillful in waiting upon one that is ailing and never unwilling to do anything that may be ordered."

—*Charaka Samhita*

"The oil lobby, perhaps the most powerful lobby on earth, is almost matched by hospital owners and doctors."
—Jimmy Carter

"Before thirty, men seek disease; after thirty, disease seeks men."
—Chinese Proverb

"The doctor sees all the weakness of the mankind, the lawyer all the wickedness, the theologian all the stupidity."
—Arthur Schopenhauer

"What fools indeed we mortals are to lavish care upon a car, with ne'er a bit of time to look after our own machinery."
—John K. Bangs

"Nature does not hurry, yet everthing is achieved."
—Lao Tzu

"The whole imposing edifice of modern medicine is like the celebrated tower of Pisa—slightly off balance."
—Charles Prince of Wales

"A fool is known by his speech, and a wise man by silence."
—Pythogoras

"Neurotic means he is not as sensible as I am, and psychotic means he's even worse than my brother-in-law."
—Karl Menninger

"Every human being is the author of his own health or disease."
—Buddha

"Knowing yourself is the beginning of all wisdom."
—Aristotle

"Every day I walk myself into a state of wellbeing and walk away from every illness. I have walked myself into my best thoughts and I know of no thought so burdensome that one cannot walk away from it. But by sitting still, and the more one sits still, the closer one comes to feeling ill…. If one keeps on walking everything will be alright."
—Soren Krickegaard

"Many ordinary illnesses are nothing but the expression of a serious dissatisfaction with life."
—Paul Tournier

"...City people shut themselves off from the processes of nature. They have air conditioning, central heating, eat hothouse vegetables, decorate with fake flowers, and even send their cats to a veterinarian to have kittens. The result is that when nature does assert itself—when illness, pain, and death loom over their petty barriers—the city dwellers are surprised and annoyed. Their attitude seems to say, 'This is all a mistake and tomorrow it will be over'—as though it were as simple as turning on a radiator to make a room warmer."
—Joseph A. Jerger

"Addiction should never be treated as a crime. It has to be treated as a health problem."
—Ralph Nader

"The biggest disease today is not leprosy or tuberculosis, but rather the feeling of being unwanted."
—Mother Teresa

"If you want others to be happy, practice compassion. If you want to be happy, practice compassion."
—Anne McCaffrey

"Cough and love cannot be hidden."
—Latin Proverb

"Sickness may be the solemn occasion of God's intervention in a person's life."
—Paul Tournier

"Our profession, after all, deals partly with guess work; we do not deal in absolutes."
—Paul Beeson

"Arise, awake and stop not until the goal is achieved."

—Swami Vivekananda

"The true index of a man's character is the health of his wife."

—Cyril Connolly

"Health is the greatest possession. Contentment is the greatest treasure. Confidence is the greatest friend. Non-being is the greatest joy."

—Lao Tzu

"We are here to add what we can to life, not to get what we can from it."

—William Osler

"The load of tomorrow added to that of yesterday, carried today, makes the strongest falter. Shut off the future as tightly as the past."

—William Osler

"Medicine, the only profession that labors incessantly to destroy the reason for its own existence."

—James Bryce

"Waste of energy, mental distress, nervous worries dog the steps of a man who is anxious about the future."

—William Osler

"The fact is that in denying the reality of sin, by giving people to understand that a fault of character is due to the malfunctioning of an endocrine gland, or by calling some impure temptation a "psychological complex," science destroys man's sense of moral responsibility. The present state of the world shows where that leads."

—Paul Tournier

"Do the difficult things while they are easy and do the great things while they are small. A journey of thousand miles must begin with a single step."

–Lao Tzu

"When I do good, I feel good. When I do bad, I feel bad."

–Abraham Lincoln

"Look to your health; and if you have it, praise God and value it next to your conscience; for health is the second blessing that we mortals are capable of, a blessing that money can't buy."

–Izaak Walton

"Halitosis is better than no breath at all."

–Anonymous

"This equilibrium is the great root from which grows all the human actions in the world, and this harmony is the universal path, which they all should pursue. Let the states of equilibrium and harmony exist in perfection, and a happy order will prevail throughout heaven and earth, and all things will be nourished and flourish."

–Confucius

"I have learned more from my mistakes than from my successes."

–Humphry Davy

"No doctor knows everything. There's a reason why it's called 'practicising' medicine."

–Anonymous

"The physician is nature's assistant."

–Galen

"You laugh, the world laughs with you. You snore, you sleep alone."

–Anthony Burgess

"To me God is psycho-neuro-immunology. My definition of God is intelligent, loving energy. God is scientific. God is light. God is darkness. God is all… Religion and science can come together… and certainly spirituality and science can come together."

—*Bernie Siegel*

"Walking uplifts the spirit. Breathe out the poisons of tension, stress and worry, breathe in the power of God. Send forth little silent prayer of goodwill towards those you meet."

—*OP Ghai*

"More people live off cancer than die from it."

—*Deepak Chopra*

"The medical scientists in India have not done anything unique or revolutionary compared to the scientists in the field of agriculture who have created successive *green* (wheat), *white* (milk) and *saffron* (oil seeds) revolutions to keep the Indian flag flying."

—*Meharban Singh*

"Any intelligent fool can make things bigger, more complex, and more violent. It takes a touch of genius and a lot of courage, to move in the oppsite direction."

—*Albert Einstein*

"A man who wastes one hour of time, has not discovered the value of life."

—*Charles Darwin*

"Humanity has but three great enemies; fever, famine and war. Of these by far the greatest, by far the most terrible is fever."

—*William Osler*

"The real knowledge is to know the extent of one's ignorance."
—Confucius

"A doctor is often more to be feared than the disease."
—French Proverb

"We all have a knack of passing the buck and blaming others, least realizing that if each one of us were to exploit his or her own full potential, no one shall ever need to be blamed for."
—Meharban Singh

"Nothing better could be preferred to God than the service to the sick and afflicted."
—CRB Sarbo

"Allergy is a term often used to give a touch of mystification to ignorance."
—Anonymous

"The most pathetic person in the world is someone who has sight, but has no vision."
—Helen Keller

"Nothing in life is to be feared, it is only to be understood. Now is the time to understand more, so that we may fear less."
—Marie Curie

"Four hundrend thousand South Africans are dying of AIDS every year. This makes the war on Iraq look like a birthday party."
—Jeremy Cronin

"Every pound of fat requires 5–6 miles of blood vessels to supply it. If a man is 30 lbs overweight, he has 25 miles of extra blood vessels with resultant strain to the heart."
—Beall

"Fat is a parasite, as we lengthen the waistline, we shorten the life line."

–Anonymous

"Cancer is a word, not a sentence."

–John Diamond

"I owe whatever success I have had to the power of setting down to the day's work and trying to do it to the best of my ability and letting the future take care of itself."

–William Osler

"Doctors cut, burn and torture the sick, then demand from them an undeserved fee for such services."

–Heraclitus

"Logic is to science what alcohol is to sex. It may stir the imagination, fire the passions and get the process underway. But the actual implementation may be found lacking and the end result may come up short."

–Anonymous

"You may not be able to read the doctor's handwriting and prescription but you'll notice his bills neatly typewritten."

–Earl Wilson

"The seed is the fetus, in other words, a true plant with its parts completely fashioned."

–Marcello Malpighi

"The studies have shown that a patient who can look out of a window during recovery from a surgery can leave the hospital much earlier than the patient who can't look out of a window. The environmental circumstances of a hospital make a difference in how well a patient recovers. For many decades we have practised medicine more for the benefit of the staff and the hospital than the benefit of the patients. And that is something that must be changed."

–David Felten

"We must, however, acknowledge, as it seems to me, that man with all his noble qualities... still bears in his bodily frame, the indelible stamp of his lowly origin."

−Charles Darwin

"When staying trim and exercising can have such a dramatic impact on the length and quality of life, just imagine the impact that vegetarian, healthy nutrition, worship, stress management, visualization, art of breathing, yoga or qigong (chi kung), spirituality and altruism could achieve."

−Alan Bryson

"Our greatest glory is not in never failing, but in getting up everytime we do."

−Confucius

"Traditionally, hospitals have been organized for doctors, for auxiliaries, for insurance companies − everybody but the patient."

−Ron Anderson

"Age appears to be the best in four things; old wood best to burn, old wine to drink, old friends to trust and old authors to read."

−Francis Bacon

"The great question that has never been answered, and which I have not yet been able to answer, despite my thirty years of research into the feminine soul is, what does a woman want?"

−Sigmund Freud

"Age is like love, it cannot be hidden."

−Thomas Dekker

"Common sense is not so common."

−Voltaire

"A hypochondriac is one who has a pill for everything except what ails him."

—Mignon McLaughlin

"The health of the people is really the foundation upon which all their happiness and all their powers as a state depend."

—Benjamin Disraeli

"The blame for producing female children (or credit for a male child) genetically rests upon the male partner because woman has no choice but to contribute only an X-chromosome."

—Meharban Singh

"Life is not merely being alive but being well."

—Martial

"So many people spend their health gaining wealth, and then they have to spend their wealth to regain their health."

—AJ Materi

"Stones grow, plants grow and live; animals grow, live and feel."

—Carl Linnaeus

"Measure your health by your symphony with morning and spring. If there is no response in you to the awakening of nature, if the prospect of any early morning walk does not banish sleep, if the warble of the first blue bird does not thrill you, know that the morning and spring of your life are past. Thus may you feel your pulse."

—Henry David Thoreau

"The dreams are true interpreters of our inclinations, but art is required to sort and understand them."

—Michel de Montaigne

"Genome is the sophisticated horoscope or *janampatri*."

–Meharban Singh

"Whatsoever you do, do with all your heart."

–Confucius

"God grant me the serenity to accept the things I cannot change, courage to change things I can, and wisdom to know the difference."

–Reinhold Niebuhr

"To live is to suffer, to survive is to find some meaning in the suffering."

–Roberta Flack

"It is not the strongest species that survive, nor the most intelligent but the one most adaptable or responsive to change."

–Charles Darwin

"Nature does nothing without a purpose."

–Aristotle

"Happiness is beneficial for the body, but it is the grief that develops powers of the mind."

–Marcel Proust

"The health of nations is more important than the wealth of nations."

–Will Durant

"The little I know, I owe to my ignorance."

–Sacha Gurtig

"Early to rise and early to bed makes a man healthy, wealthy and dead!"

–James Thurber

"Perfect health, like perfect beauty, is a rare thing, and so, it seems, is perfect disease."
    —Peter Mere Latham

"I have never met a man so ignorant that I couldn't learn something from him."
    —Galileo Galilei

"Truth in all its kind is most difficult to win and truth in medicine is the most difficult of all."
    —Peter Mere Latham

"Common sense in medicine is the master workman."
    —Peter Mere Latham

"Errors like straws upon the surface flow, he who would search for pearls, must dive below."
    —John Dryden

"Ignorance is like knowledge, there is no end to it."
    —Anonymous

"Man is a creature composed of countless millions of cells; a microbe is composed of only one, yet throughout the ages the two have been in ceaseless conflict."
    —AB Christie

"As arteries go hard, the heart goes soft."
    —HL Mencken

"Old people have fewer diseases than the young, but their diseases never leave them."
    —Hippocrates

"Medicine is a noble profession but a damn bad business."
    —Humphrey Ralleston

"The most beautiful things in the world cannot be seen or even touched. They must be felt with the heart."

–Helen Keller

"Just like finding a suitable spouse, finding the right physician is no less a daunting task in the modern society."

–Meharban Singh

"I have seen good deeds done by men with ugly faces, and flowers grow in stony places, so I trust both."

–AL Cochrane

"While medicine is a science, in many particulars it cannot be exact, so baffling are the varying results of varying conditions of human life."

–Charles Horace Mayo

"My life is in the hands of any fool who makes me lose my temper. What matters is not to add years to your life but to add life to your years."

–Alexis Carrel

"Anatomy is to physiology as geography is to history, it describes the theatre of events."

–Jean Fernel

"Man is the only animal that laughs and weeps; for he is the only animal that is struck with the difference between what things are, and what they ought to be."

–Hazlitt

"All truly great thoughts are conceived while walking."

–Friedrich Nietzche

"The less you open your heart to others, the more your heart suffers."

–Deepak Chopra

"The heart is wiser than the intellect."

–JG Holland

"Happy is the man who has broken the chains which hurt the mind and has given up worrying once and for all."

–Tristia

"To know that we know what we know, and that what we don't know we do not know, that is true knowledge."

–Confucius

"Drink because you are happy, but never because you are miserable."

–GK Chesterton

"The fate of a nation has often depended on the good or bad digestion of a Prime Minister."

–Voltaire

"Oh health, the blessing of the rich, the riches of the poor, who can buy thee at too dear a rate, since there is no enjoying this world without thee."

–Ben Jonson

"Every patient carries her or his own doctor within."

–Albert Schweitzer

"To handle yourself, use your head, to handle others, use your heart. The pain of the mind is worse than the pain of the body."

–Syrus

"For all the happiness, mankind can gain, is not in pleasure but in freedom from pain."

–John Dryden

"We should learn from childhood not to hold grudges. Children often fight when they play together but they quickly make up and their fights don't deteriorate into bitter feuds."

–Joseph Wechsberg

"Every form of addiction is bad, no matter whether it is narcotic, alcohol or morphine or idealism."

–Carl Gustav Jung

"Life is an incurable disease."

–Abraham Cowley

"Disease is war with the laws of our being, and all war, as a great General has said, is hell."

–Lewis G. Janes

"Be not slow to visit the sick."

–Ecclesiastes

"A little learning is a dangerous thing."

–Ben Franklin

"Get people better and they will send more new patients to you that you can treat."

–George Goodheart

"True science teaches, above all, to doubt and to be ignorant."

–Miguel de Unamuno

"As it takes two to make a quarrel, so it takes two to make a disease, the microbe and its host."

–Charles V. Chapin

"Microbes are not as important because terrain is everything!"

–Louis Pasteur

"People are more scared of pain than death. And most people would do anything to avoid pain but not so much for gaining pleasure."

–Anonymous

"The lofty objective of "Health for All" cannot be achieved merely by a slogan, unless we ensure, Education for All, Food for All, Homes for All, Safe Drinking Water for All, Jobs for All and above all Dignity for All."

–Meharban Singh

"One thousand Americans stop smoking every day—by dying."

–Anonymous

"The word "health" is beautiful. It comes from the same root as the word "whole". Health, healing, whole, holy— they all come from the same root. Mind is a disease, a holy or healthy man lives without mind."

–Osho

"First thing a child has to do when he is born is to breathe in. And the last thing when a man dies will be to breathe out. Each moment you breathe in, you are reborn, each moment you breathe out you are dead because breath is life. That's why Hindus have called it *prana: Prana* means life. Breath is life."

–Osho

"Always remember that worst things in your life have within them the seeds of the best."

–Joe Kogel

"Words can kill as well as heal."

–Bernard Lown

"A man who works with his hands is a laborer; a man who works with his hands and brain is a craftsman; but a man who works with his hands and his brain and his heart is an artist."

–Louis Nizer

"I have the conviction that when physiology will be far enough advanced, the poet, the philosopher and the physiologist will all understand each other."

—Claude Bernard

"Medicine sometimes snatches away health, sometimes gives it."

—Ovid Tristia

"Our body is in a dynamic equilibrium, being constantly broken down and continuously replaced without our knowledge and perception. The skin replaces itself once a month, the stomach lining every five days, the liver every six weeks and the skeleton every three months. Every minute nearly 300 million cells die and are replaced by new ones. Almost 98 percent atoms in our body get exchanged within a period of one year."

—Scientific Fact

"If you do not want to catch cold, fall in love."

—Popular Saying

"Health, happiness and success are beyond our grasp without self-love, confidence and self-esteem."

—Gloria Steinem

"Man is ill because he is never still."

—Paracelsus

"The first half of our lives is ruined by our parents and second half by our children."

—Clarence Darrow

"Sow a thought, reap an action
  Sow an action, reap a habit
  Sow a habit, reap a character
  Sow a character, reap a destiny."

—Chinese Proverb

"If your body is straight, your channels will be straight. If your channels are straight, your mind will be straight."

—Tibetan Saying

"If I were a medical man, I shall prescribe a holiday to every patient who considered his work important."

—Bertrand Russel

"It is amazing that only 5% of the genetic material in DNA is used for its complicated coding, self-repair and production of RNA, leaving 95% doing nothing that science can account for. There is thus tremendous untapped and unknown potential."

—Scientific Fact

"My doctor gave me six months to live but when I couldn't pay the bill, he gave me six months more."

—Walter Matthau

"All the violence, fear and suffering that exist in the world comes from grasping the self. What use is this great evil monster to you? If you do not let go of the self, there will never be an end to your suffering. Just as if you do not release a flame from your hand, you can't stop it from burning your hand."

—Shantideva

"We are motivated in life by two overriding drives, to procreate and to survive. It seems pain and pleasure motivates our actions. Most people will do everything to avoid pain than to gain pleasure."

—Sigmund Freud

"Someone said to me, "I hope you live to see all your dreams fulfilled." I replied, 'I hope not, because if all my dreams are fulfilled, I'm dead.' It's unfulfilled dreams that keep you alive."

—Robert Schuller

"Doctors will have more lives to answer for the next world than even we Generals."

—*Napolean Bonaparte*

"When we are unable to find tranquillity within ourselves, it is useless to seek it elsewhere."

—*La Rochefoucauld*

"What lies behind us and what is before us are tiny matters compared to what lies within us."

—*Ralph Waldo Emerson*

"A busy mind is a sick mind, a quiet mind is a healthy mind; but a still mind is a divine mind."

—*Indian Saying*

"The modern sympathy with invalids is morbid. Illness of any kind is hardly a thing to be encouraged in others."

—*Oscar Wilde*

"Great spirits have always engendered violent opposition from mediocre minds."

—*Albert Einstein*

"Birth, copulation and death; that's all the facts when you come to brass tacks."

—*TS Eliot*

"Disease is the retribution of outraged nature."

—*Isadora Duncan*

"The female species of animals and insects have been tormenting the human race from times immemorial. It is the female *Anophelese, Aedes aegypti* and *Culex* that transmit malaria, dengue fever, chikungunya, filaria and Japanese encephalitis. It is the female genres of spiders that cause lethal bites to the humans while males are meek and docile. And the female tyranny continues even when the human race is more and more evolved. We should actually talk of male agony and not of female bigotry."

–Meharban Singh

"Old is gold was coined as a tribute to physicians."

–Meharban Singh

"Familiarity breeds contempt – and children."

–Mark Twain

"All happy families resemble one another; every unhappy family is unhappy in its own way."

–Leo Tolstoy

"There is no great genius without madness."

–Aristotle

"Genius is one percent inspiration and ninety nine percent perspiration."

–TA Edison

"To be good only to yourself is to be good for nothing."

–Voltaire

"Grey hair is a sign of age, not of wisdom."

–Greek Proverb

"Look to your health, and if you have it, praise God, and value it next to a good conscience; for health is the second blessing we mortals are capable of; a blessing that money cannot buy."

–Izzak Walton

"To save a man's life against his will is the same as killing him."

–Horace

"If ignorance is bliss, why aren't there many happy people?"

–S. White

"Strange how much you've got to know, before you know how little you know."

–Anonymous

"To be conscious that you are ignorant is a great step to knowledge."

–Benjamin Disraeli

"Life is a jigsaw puzzle with most of the pieces missing."

–Anonymous

"Love's like the measles – all the worse when it comes late in life."

–D. Jerrold

"A hospital bed is a parked taxi with the meter running."

–Groucho Marx

"What is human, is immortal."

–Bulwer-Lytton

"Little deeds of kindness, little words of love, help to make earth happy like the heaven above."

–Julia F. Carney

"I shall pass through this world but once. If, therefore, there be any kindness I can show, or any good deed I can do, let me do it now; let me not defer it or neglect it, for I shall not pass this way again."

–E de Grellet

"If I can stop one heart from breaking, I shall not live in vain. If I can ease one life the aching or cool one pain or help one fainting robbin, unto his nest again, I shall not live in vain."

–Emily Dickinson

"Be noble in every thought; and in every deed."
–Longfellow

"Nature gave man two ends – one to sit on and one to think with. Ever since then man's success or failure has been dependent on the one he used most."
–GR Kirkpatrick

"I never did a day's work in my life, it was all fun."
–Thomas Edison

"There are no illegitimate children—only illegitimate parents."
–Leon R Yankwich

"Parents learn a lot from their children about coping with life."
–M. Spark

"The world is beautiful but has a disease called Man."
–Friedrich Nietzsche

"No human being is constituted to know the truth, the whole truth, and nothing but the truth; and even the best of men must be content with fragments, with partial glimpses, never the full fruition."
–William Osler

"Common sense nerve fibers are seldom medullated before forty—they are never seen even with a microscope before twenty."
–William Osler

"As to your method of work, I have a single bit of advice, which I give with the earnest conviction of its paramount influence in any success which may have attended my efforts in life—Take no thought for the morrow. Live neither in the past nor in the future, but let each day's work, absorb your entire energies, and satisfy your wildest ambition."
–William Osler

"I have two fixed ideas...The first is the comparative usefulness of men above forty years of age... My second fixed idea is the uselessness of men above sixty years of age, and the incalculable benefit it would be in commercial, political and in professional life if, as a matter of course, men stopped work at this age."

−William Osler

"Each case has its lesson—a lesson that may be, but is not always learnt, for clinical wisdom is not the equivalent of experience. A man who has seen 500 cases of pneumonia may not have the understanding of the disease which comes with an intelligent study of a score of cases, so different are knowledge and wisdom, which, as the poet truly says, 'far from being one have oft-times no connection'."

−William Osler

"One of the first essentials in securing a good natured equanimity is not to expect too much of the people amongst whom you dwell."

−William Osler

"Experience in the true sense of the term does not come to all with years, or with increasing opportunities. Growth in the acquisition of facts is not necessarily associated with development. Many grow through life as the crystal, by simple accretion, and at fifty possess, to vary the figure, the unicellular mental blastoderm with which they started."

−William Osler

"I have had three personal ideals. *One* to do the day's work well and not to bother about tomorrow... the *second* ideal has been to act the golden rule, as far as in me lay, towards my professional brethren and towards the patients committed to my care. And the *third* has been to cultivate such a measure of equanimity as would enable me to bear success with humility, the affection of my friends without pride and to be ready when the day of sorrow and grief came to meet it with the courage befitting a man."

–William Osler

"We are all born with a fixed quota of food and allotted number of breaths. It is in our own hands to finish our quota earlier by eating excessively or breathing fast. The best mantra to live long is to eat less and eat right, breathe slow and breathe right."

–Meharban Singh

"The philosophies of one age have become the absurdities of the next, and the foolishness of yesterday has become the wisdom of tomorrow."

–William Osler

"Mankind has survived all catastrophes; it will also survive modern medicine."

–Gerhard Kocher

"A wise man should consider that health is the greatest of human blessings, and learn how by his own thought, derive benefit from his illnesses."

–Hippocrates

"Health and wealth create beauty."

–English Proverb

"Pomegranate a day, keeps the cardiologist away."

–Popular Saying

"However discordant or troubled you have been during the day, do not go to sleep until you have restored your mental balance, until your faculties are poised and your mind is serene."

–Orison Swett Marden

"Some people bear three kinds of troubles—all they ever had, all they have now, and all they expect to have."
—Edward Everett Hale

"Fear is an acid which is pumped into one's atmosphere. It causes mental, moral and spiritual asphyxiation and sometimes death, death to energy and all growth."
—Horace Fletcher

"Mirth is God's medicine, everybody ought to bathe in it. Grim care, moroseness, anxiety — all the rust of life — ought to be scoured off by the oil of mirth."
—Oliver Wendell Holmes

"Medicine is a social science, and politics is nothing more than medicine in a larger scale."
—Rudolph Virchow

"On any given day, your patients and their families will treat you like God. As long as you don't believe it, it's okay. And if you do, it's the beginning of the end."
—Frank Spencer

"Iron rusts from disuse, stagnant water loses its purity, and in cold weather water becomes frozen, even so does inaction sap the vigour of the mind."
—Leonardo da Vinci

"The best six doctors anywhere and no one can deny it are sunshine, water, rest, air, exercise and diet. These six will gladly attend to you, if only you are willing. Your mind they'll mend and charge you not a shilling."
—Thomas Fuller

"Advances in medicine and agriculture have saved vastly more lives than have been lost in all the wars in history."
—Carl Sagan

"Medicine is my lawful wife and literature my mistress, when I get tired of one, I spend the night with the other."

–Anton Chekhov

"He's is a fool that makes his doctor his heir."

–Benjamin Franklin

"I love doctors and hate their medicine."

–Walt Whitmans

"If you are physically sick, you can elicit the interest of a battery of physicians, but if you are mentally sick, you are lucky if the Janitor comes around."

–Martin H. Fischer

"Life is short, the art long, opportunity fleeting, experience treacherous, judgement difficult. The physician must be ready, not only to do his duty himself, but also to secure the cooperation of the patient, of the attendant and of externals."

–Hippocrates

"The best mantra to promote health and mental poise is to accept and say 'haarmaani' (I am at fault) in order to maintain harmony."

–BK Shivani

"Philosophy is the sister of medicine."

–Tertullian

18

Motherhood and Mothercraft

"Where have I come from, where did you pick me up; the baby asked its mother. She answered half-crying, half-laughing and clasping the baby to her breast. You were hidden in my heart as its desire, my darling. You were in the dolls of my childhood games, and when with clay I made the image of my god every morning, I made and unmade you then."

—Rabindranath Tagore

"A woman with a child, if it be a male, has a good color, but if a female, she has a bad color."

—Hippocrates

"Mothers love their children more than fathers, because parenthood cost the mother more trouble."

—Aristotle

"A mother exceedeth a thousand fathers in the right to reverence."

—Manu

"The duties of motherhood requires qualities and attributes which man does not possess. The art of bringing up children of the race is her special forte and sole prerogative. Without her care the race will become extinct…"

—Mahatma Gandhi

"A baby is an inestimable blessing and bother."

–Mark Twain

"Birthday: The only day in life, when your mother smiled when you cried—otherwise whenever you cried, she also cried."

–APJ Abdul Kalam

"Making the decision to have a child is momentous. It is as if to decide forever to have your heart go walking outside your body."

–Elizabeth Stone

"Parents influence their offspring's eugenically before conception, physiologically during pregnancy and socially after birth. Mother's contribution and commitment is far greater than father's."

–RC Mitchell

"Gender equality and well-being of children go hand in hand. When women are empowered to live full and productive lives they let children prosper. When women are denied equal opportunity within a society, children suffer."

–The State of World's Children, UNICEF 2007

"The nature has desired the provision that infants be fed upon their mother's milk. They find their food and mother at the same time. It is a complete nourishment for them both for their body and soul."

–Rabindranath Tagore

"Any woman can give birth to a child, that is a simple biological process. But to be a good mother needs great art, understanding and compassion."

–Anonymous

"The education of a child begins with conception."

–Mahatma Gandhi

"There is no velvet as soft as a mother's lap. No rose as lovely as her smile. No path as flowery as that imprinted with her footsteps."

–Archibald Thompson

"When a child is born, a mother is also born. The ordinary woman achieves the exalted status of a mother."

–Meharban Singh

"...... There is no tool for development more effective than the education of girls."

–Kofi A. Annan

"Mother is the name for God in the lips and hearts of little children."

–William H. Thackeray

"If ever I get a chance, I should love to be reborn just to have the ecstacy of being reared by the kind and caring mother."

–W. Oscar

"Investing in girls education today...... is a strategy that will protect the rights of all children to quality education.... and a strategy that will jump-start all other development goals."

–The State of the World's Children, UNICEF 2004

"For the hand that rocks the cradle, is the hand that rules the world."

–WS Ross

"Men are what their mothers made them."

–Emerson

"Where women are revered, there the gods reside. Where women are not revered, all actions become futile."

–Manusmriti

"God could not be everywhere, therefore he created mothers."

—Talmud

Society should see parenting as a public health issue and help parents to bring their children up feeling loved. We have birthing classes but no parenting classes."

—Bernie Siegel

"Communities and countries, and ultimately the world are only as strong as the health of their women."

—Michelle Obama

"Perfect love sometimes does not come until the first grandchild."

—Welsh Proverb

"When grandparents enter the door, discipline flies out the window."

—Ogden Nash

"Grandparents are God's way of compensating us for growing old."

—Mary H. Waldrip

"Grandmas hold or tiny hands for just a little while, but our hearts forever."

—Author Unknown

Oaths and Codes

"Dedicate yourself entirely to helping the sick, even though this be at the cost of your own life. Never harm the sick, not even in thought. Endeavor always to perfect your knowledge. Treat no woman except in the presence of their husbands. The physician should observe all the rules of good dress and good conduct. As soon as he is with a patient, he should concern himself in word and thought with nothing but the sufferer's case. He must not speak outside the house of anything that takes place in the patient's house. He must not speak to a patient of his possible death if so doing he hurts the patient or anyone else. In the sights of gods, you are to pledge yourself to this. May the gods help you if you follow this rule. Otherwise, may the gods be against you."

—Manu's Code of Conduct for Physicians

"I swear by Apollo, the physician, by Asclepius, by Health, by Hygieia and Panaceia and by all the gods and goddesses, making them my witness, that I will carry out, according to my ability and judgement, this oath and this indenture. To hold my teacher in this art equal to my parents, to make him partner in my livelihood, when he is in need of money to share mine with him, to consider his family as my own brothers, and to teach them this art, if they want to learn it, without fee or indenture....

I will use treatment to help the sick according to my ability and judgement, but never with a view to injury or wrongdoing. Neither will I administer a poison to anybody when asked to do so, nor will I suggest such a course. Similarly I will not give to a woman a pessary to cause abortion.

I will keep pure and holy both my life and my art... In whatsoever houses I enter, I will enter to help the sick, and I will abstain from all intentional wrongdoing and harm, especially from abusing the bodies of man or woman, bond or free. And whatsoever I shall see or hear in the course of my profession in my intercourse with men, if it be what should not be published abroad, I will never divulge, holding such things to be holy secrets.

Now if I carry out this oath and break it not, may I gain forever reputation among all men for my life and for my art, but if I transgress it and forswear myself, may the opposite befall me."

—Hippocratic Oath

"The teacher then should instruct the disciple in the presence of the sacred fire, Brahmanas (Brahmins) and physicians... Thou shalt behave and act without arrogance, with care and attention and with undistracted mind, humility, constant reflection and ungrudging obedience. Acting either at my behest or otherwise, thou shalt conduct thyself for the achievement of thy teacher's purposes alone, to the best of thy abilities. If thou desires success, wealth and fame as a physician and heaven after death, thou shalt pray for the welfare of all creatures beginning with the cows and Brahmanas......

Day and night, however, thou mayest be engaged, thou shalt endeavor for the relief of patients with all thy heart and soul. Thou shalt not desert or injure thy patient for the sake of thy life or thy living. Thou shalt not commit adultery even in thought. Thou shalt be modest in thy attire and appearance. Thou shouldst not be a drunkard or a sinful man nor shouldst thou associate with the abettors of crimes. Thou shouldst speak words that are gentle, pure and righteous, pleasing, worthy, true, wholesome, and moderate...

Thou shalt act always with a view to the acquisition of knowledge and fullness of equipment... While entering the patient's house, thou shalt be accompanied by a man who is known to the patient and who has his permission to enter; and thou shalt be well-clad, bent of head, self-possessed, and conduct thyself only after repeated considerations. Having entered, thy speech, mind, intellect and senses shall be entirely devoted to no other thought than that of being helpful to the patient and of things concerning only him.

Even knowing that the patient's span of life has come to its close, it shall not be mentioned by thee there, where if so done, it would cause shock to the patient or to others. There is no limit at all to the Science of Life, Medicine. So thou shouldst apply thyself to it with diligence. Thou shouldst conduct thyself properly with the gods, sacred fire, Brahmanas, the guru, the aged, the scholars and the preceptors. To the teacher that has spoken thus, the disciple should say, 'Amen'."

–Charaka Oath

"... Not for the self, not for the fulfilment of any wordly material desire or gain; but solely for the good of humanity, I will treat my patients and excel all..."

–Charaka Oath

(Abridged oath administered at AIIMS graduation ceremony)

"The eternal providence has appointed me to watch over the life and health of thy creatures. May the love of my art actuate me at all time, may neither avarice or miserliness, nor thirst for glory or for a great reputation engage my mind, for the enemies of truth and philanthropy could easily deceive me and make me forgetful of my lofty aim of doing good to thy children. May I never see the patient anything but a fellow creature in pain. Grant me the strength, time and opportunity always to correct what I have acquired, always to extend its domain, for knowledge is immense and the spirit of man can extend indefinately to enrich itself daily with new requirements.

Today thous can discover his errors of yesterday and tomorrow thou can obtain a new light on what you think yourself sure of today. Oh God, thou has appointed me to watch over the life and death of thy creatures, here am I ready for my vocation and now I turn unto my calling."

–Moses ben Maimonides Oath

"I solemnly pledge myself to consecrate my life to the service of humanity. Even under threat, I will not use my medical knowledge contrary to the laws of humanity. I will maintain utmost respect for human life from the time of conception. I will not permit consideration of religion, nationality, race, party politics or social standing to intervene between my duty and my patient. I will practice my profession with conscience and dignity. The health of my patient will be my first consideration. I will not permit consideration of religion, nationality, race, party-politics or social standing to intervene between my duty and my patient. I will respect the secrets, which are confided in me. I will give to my teachers the respect and gratitude which is their due. I will maintain by all means in my power, the honor and noble traditions of medical profession. I will treat my colleagues with all due respect and dignity. I make these promises solemnly, freely and upon my honor."

–Medical Council of India Oath

"I solemnly pledge myself to consecrate my life to the service of humanity. I will give my teachers the respect and gratitude which is their due. I will practice my profession with conscience and dignity. The health of my patients will be my first consideration. I will respect the secrets, which are confided in me even after the patient has died. I will not permit the consideration of religion, nationality, race, party-politics or social standing to intervene between my duty and my patient. I will maintain the utmost respect for the human life from the time of conception. Even under threat; I will not use any medical knowledge contrary to the laws of humanity. I will maintain by all the means in my power to honor the noble traditions of the medical profession. My colleagues will be my brothers and sisters. I make these promises solemnly, freely and upon my honor."

—The Declaration of Geneva

I shall maintain the highest standards of professional conduct, to practise uninfluenced by motive of profit. To use caution in divulging discoveries or new techniques of treatment. To certify or testify only those matters with which the doctor has personal experience. To ensure that any act or advice that could weaken physical or mental resistance of an individual must be used only in the interest of that individual.

Always remember the obligation of preserving life. The patient has owed complete loyalty, and all the resources of medical science should be harnessed. Whenever a treatment or examination is beyond the capacity of the doctor, the advice of another doctor should be sought. A doctor must always preserve absolute secrecy concerning all he knows about a patient, because of the confidence trusted in him. Emergency care is a humanitarian duty which must be given, unless it is clear that there are others better able to give it.

A doctor must behave to his colleagues as he would have them behave toward him. A doctor must not entice patients from his colleagues. A doctor must observe the principles of the Declaration of Geneva.

The unethical practices include any self-advertisement except as expressly authorized in a national code of ethics, collaboration in any form of medical services in which the doctor does not have professional independence and receipt of any money in connection with services rendered to a patient other than a proper professional fee, even if the patient is aware of it."

—International Code of Medical Ethics

20

Perinatal Medicine

"Just as the child is not a mini-adult, the neonate is not a mini-child."

—Meharban Singh

"Health and wellbeing of a fetus is dependent upon the health and nutrition of the mother (not the father!) because she is both the seed as well as the soil wherein baby is nurtured for nine months."

—Meharban Singh

"Nothing is more humanized than feeding the babies with human milk."

—Meharban Singh

"The art of newborn care should not be sacrificed at the altar of technology. Art and science should provide an harmonious blend to ensure holistic care."

—Meharban Singh

"Diagnosis of a neonatal disorder is based more on the nature of predisposing and associated conditions and antecedent events rather than the clinical manifestations at the time of presentation."

—Meharban Singh

"... 61 percent of all deformities in newborn infants and 88 percent of all stillbirths must be attributed to the effects of medicaments."

—W. Chr

"Newborn screening is a public health intervention that involves a simple blood test used to identify many life-threatening genetic illnesses before any symptoms begin."

–Lucille Roybal-Allard

"Neonates constitute the foundation of a nation and mothers are its pillars. And no sensible government can afford to neglect their needs and rights."

–UNICEF

"The enhancement of neonatal and infant survival is truly the key to the success of family welfare program and stabilization of population dynamics, which is a major public health issue in developing countries."

–V. Ramalingaswami

"There is no indicator in human biology, which tells us as much about the past events and the future trajectory of life as the weight of the baby at birth."

–V. Ramalingaswami

"Every birth must be viewed as a medical emergency. We should be prepared to meet the challenge of 26 million medical emergencies every year in our country."

–Meharban Singh

"Most problems in healthy term newborn babies are minor, physiological or developmental and without any clinical significance. But when a newborn baby is genuinely sick, he is likely to be very sick and cannot be managed on an ambulatory basis."

–Meharban Singh

"We do know how to treat hyperbilirubinemia in the newborn but we do not know when to treat it because there is as yet no single test that can identify the level of bilirubin which is dangerous to the brain."

–Meharban Singh

"Around 96% of global neonatal deaths occur in developing countries. There is a need to build global opinion in favor of newborn care as the most urgent key health priority."

—World Health Organization

"Milk is not only species specific, it is baby specific. The milk of a mother is best suited to serve the biological needs of her own baby."

—Meharban Singh

"The physical and mental health of mother before, during and after pregnancy has a profound effect on the status and survival of the fetus in-utero and infant after birth."

—Anonymous

"Newborn infant is a "blank page" on which environment and education write this or that story of the individual's life."

—J J Rousseau

"Seeds of cerebral palsy are sown in the perinatal period."

—Meharban Singh

"There has been no consistent decrease in the incidence of cerebral palsy in the last 1–2 decades despite advances in perinatal monitoring and management. Are deaths being converted into disability?"

—Anonymous

"The mental apparatus of the coming generation is developed in the womb and the time to begin supplementation is before conception. A normal brain cannot be made without an adequate supply of omega-3 fatty acids, and there may be no later opportunity to repair the effects of omega-3 fatty acid deficiency once the nervous system is formed."

—William E. Connor

"Mother's milk contains about thirty times more brain-essential DHA than cow's milk."

–Scientific Fact

"The seeds of neonatal morbidity are sown in the labor room."

–Meharban Singh

"Let us not allow the technology to further dehumanize neonatology. We must treat babies not only with our heads but also with our hearts. And the narrow focus on hi-tech medical rescues in NICUs should give way to compassionate acts of social interventions for global benefits for all rather than narrow gains for a few."

–Meharban Singh

"The human fetus has been likened to a spaceman; passive, insulated and preserved from stimuli, which is only half the truth. On the contrary, one could think of the mammalian embryo as a hitch-hiker with a large pack on his back getting into a rather small car. He is a friendly fellow who chatters away all the time and is prepared to do so driving. If given half the chance he takes you off your route and tells when and where he would like to get out."

–Geoffery Dawes

Plea of a baby at birth

"I have come from an extremely warm, clean, quiet and comfortable abode. Protect me at birth from microbes and cold.

I am wet and naked, dry me, cover me and place me under a heater.

I don't know how to smile, let me announce my arrival by a cry.

Don't hurt me but gently clean my windpipe to let me cry.

Don't give me injections but give me a breath to save my life.
I have been swimming all through in the womb.
Don't be in a hurry to bathe me in the labor room."

–*Meharban Singh*

Prayer of a premature baby

"I came too early, I came too light.
From the warm womb, to the cold room,
struggling for breath, trying to survive.
Hungry for food, to keep the brain alive.

The invisible enemy, threatens through you.
And the yellow pigment, ever ready to cripple.
Lungs too stiff to get oxygen to blood,
if only you care, I need special care.

Brain bleeds with strain, blood channels too fragile.
Be gentle, be kind, be warm for a while.
By your thoughtful care, given this start
I may be Winston Churchill, I may be Bonaparte."

–*ON Bhakoo*

"The newborn baby has a limited capacity to express specific clinical manifestations of a disease process. He is likely to manifest with identical nonspecific stereotyped responses to a variety of disorders."

–*Meharban Singh*

"Fetus is fully aware and perceptive in the womb. The uterine blood flow provides a sonorous music akin to a waterfall while tick-tack of the maternal heart beats provides him the soothing beats of a cuckoo-clock. No wonder we are all fascinated by the sight and sound of a waterfall which is reminiscent of our in-utero abode."

–*Meharban Singh*

"Genes provide a general recipe for making a human being, but the human being is determined by the ingredients provided by the mother."

—David Barker

"Apart from physical connection, there is an ethereal or spiritual bond between the mother and her baby in the womb. Every emotion experienced by the mother is transmitted as vibrations and vibes to her baby. Your thoughts and perceptions have a profound effect on your unborn baby—Be meditative and have positive and vibrant thoughts of love, peace and hope to touch the soul of your baby."

—Meharban Singh

"Newborn indeed is a 'seed', endowed with immense potentiality. You can't do anything to alter its genome but you can provide optimal nurturing, nutrition, safe environment and global health care to unfold myriads of human capabilities to help him evolve as a robust citizen of the society.

—Meharban Singh

21

Physicians and Medical Students

"The medical student must exhibit a calm and generous disposition, besides being virtuous and of noble mind. He must be tolerant of others and exhibit patience and perseverance in his academic pursuits. Although of sharp intellect, he must be both rational and modest. He should possess a pleasant appearance and good looks with a well-proportioned body which should be free from physical defects or any obvious diseases. Above all, he must be compassionate. He must exhibit deep interest in the art and science of healing. He must use his intelligence to discuss facts about the disease and to understand the clinical significance of symptoms. Such knowledge he must use not only for his own intellectual enrichment, but also for acquiring requisite skills in practical management. He must be humble and loyal to his teachers and instructors. He should be free from any addictions, greed, arrogance and intolerance."

–Charak Samhita

"Nature, Time and Patience are three great physicians."

–HG Bohn

"My doctor is nice; every time I see him, I'm ashamed of what I think of doctors in general."

–Mignon McLaughlin

"In nothing do men more nearly approach the gods than in giving health to men."

—Cicero

"Every disease is a physician."

—Irish Proverb

"To be a doctor, then, means much more than to dispense pills or to patch up or repair torn flesh and shattered minds. To be a doctor is to be an intermediary between man and God."

—Felix Marti-Ibanez

"Oh God! protect us, both teacher and student. Take adequate care of us both. Provide us power and the knowledge attained be a beacon of light. We be unbeatable in knowledge and both be friendly for the whole life. And enmity should never develop within ourselves. Let there be peace! peace! peace!"

—Upanishads

"Physician heal thyself."

—Bible

"I often say, a great doctor kills more people than a great General."

—GW Leibniz

"I know nothing more laughable than a doctor who does not die of old age."

—Voltaire

"Doctors assist us to come safely into the world and comfortably out of it, and during life to protect the well and care for the sick and disabled."

—Thomas McKeown

"A doctor's reputation is made by the number of eminent men who die under his care."

–George Bernard Shaw

"A physician without knowledge of astrology has no right to call himself a physician."

–Hippocrates

"Medicine is perhaps the oldest of the technologies. It represents a skill based on a body of knowledge, daily growing in extent and in exactitude, and applied to the limited end of alleviating human suffering."

–George White Pickering

"The best physicians are Dr Diet, Dr Quiet, and Dr Merryman."

–French Proverb

"One has a greater sense of intellectual degradation after an interview with a doctor than from any human experience."

–Alice James

"But nothing is not estimable than a physician who, having studied nature from his youth, knows the properties of the human body, the diseases which assail it, the remedies which will benefit it, exercises his art with caution, and pays equal attention to the rich and poor.

–Voltaire

"Physicians are like wine, they mature with age."

–Meharban Singh

"No physician is really good before he has killed one or two patients."

–Hindu Proverb

"Don't live in a town where there are no doctors."

–Jewish Proverb

"People are afraid of authority figures and doctors are authority figures."

—Martha Beck

"God and the doctor we alike adore
  But only when in danger, not before;
  The danger o'er, both are alike requited,
  God is forgotten, and the doctor slighted."

—Robert Owen

"Orthodox medicine has not found an answer to your complaint. However, luckily for you, I happen to be a quack."

—Richter

"As long as men are liable to die and are desirous to live, a physician will be made fun of, but he will be well paid."

—La Bruyere

"A physician is obligated to consider more than a diseased organ, more even than the whole man—he must view the man in his world."

—Harvey Cushing

"But nothing is more estimable than a physician, who having studied nature from his youth, knows the properties of the human body, the diseases which assail it, the remedies which will benefit, exercises his art with caution, and pays equal attention to the rich and the poor."

—Voltaire

"The superior doctor prevents sickness; The mediocre doctor attends to impending sickness; The inferior doctor treats actual sickness;"

—Chinese Proverb

"The ideal pediatrician must have genuine interest and love for children. He should approach children as children (not patients!) in a playful and friendly manner, with tact, gentleness, compassion and concern."

—Meharban Singh

"It is a good thing for a physician to have prematurely grey hair and itching piles. The first makes him appear to know more than he does, and the second gives him an expression of concern which the patient interprets as being on his behalf."

—Benson A. Cannon

"Every day doctors have to deal with people who are worn out and unable to stand up to the life they lead. They generally assert that it is impossible to alter the way they live, and sincerely believe that their overwork is the product of circumstances, whereas it is bound up with their own intimate problems. It is ambition, fear of the future, love of money, jealousy, or social injustice that makes men strive and overwork, invent all sorts of unnecessary tasks, keep late hours, take too little sleep, take insufficient holidays, or use their holidays badly. Their minds are overtense, so that at night they cannot sleep and by day they doubly fatigue themselves at their work."

—Paul Tournier

"In a sick room, ten cents' worth of human understanding equals ten dollars' worth of medical science."

—Martin H. Fischer

"The patient does not care about your science; what he wants to know is, can you cure him?"

—Martin H. Fischer

"The world needs caring and concerned physicians and not merely curing and commercial robots."

—Meharban Singh

"Some patients, though conscious that their condition is perilous, recover their health simply through their contentment with the goodness of the physician."

–Hippocrates

"Doctors make the very worst patients."

–Popular Saying

"Honor a physician with the honor due unto him for the uses which ye may have of him; for the Lord hath created him."

–Ecclesiastes

"Next to finding one's spouse, finding the right physician is one of the most daunting tasks we face in life."

–Alan Bryson

"Any physician who advertises a positive cure for any disease, who issues nostrum testimonials, who sells his services of a secret remedy, or who diagnoses and treats his mail patients he has never seen, is a quack."

–Samuel Hopkins Adams

"An inquiring, analytical mind; an unquenchable thirst for new knowledge; and a heartfelt compassion for the ailing— these are prominent traits among the committed clinicians who have preserved the passion for medicine."

–Lois DeBakey

"Men who are occupied in the restoration of health to other men, by the joint exertion of skill and humanity, are above all the great on the earth. They even partake of divinity, since to preserve and renew is almost as noble as to create."

–Voltaire

"The education of the doctor which goes on after he has his degree is, after all, the most important part of his education."

–John Shaw Billings

"The mark of professional people is that they embody a set of principles. They understand them. They literally "stand under them", they are able to remove their own needs and focus their entire attention on what needs to be done, for as long as is necessary, doing it for its own sake, not for any other reason."

—Plato

"The wider and freer a man's general education, the better practitioner he is likely to be."

—William Osler

"A certain doctor defines a doctor to be a man who writes prescriptions till the patient either dies or is cured by nature."

—Peter Shaw

"The medical student begins with the patient, continues with the patient, and ends his studies with the patient, using books and lectures as tools, as means to an end."

—William Osler

"Learn as if you were to live for ever, live as if you were to die tomorrow."

—Isidone

"It behaves every person who purposes to give himself to the care of others, seriously to consider the four following things: *First*, that he must one day give an account to the Supreme Judge of all the lives entrusted to his care. *Second*, that all his skill and knowledge and energy, as they have been given to him by God, so they should be exercised for His glory and the good of mankind, and not for mere gain or ambition. *Third*, and not more beautifully than truly, let him reflect that he has undertaken the care of no mean creature; for, in order that he may estimate the value, the greatness of the human race, the only begotten Son of God became himself a man and thus ennobled it with His divine dignity, and far more than this, died to redeem it. And *fourth*, that the doctor being himself a mortal human being, should be diligent and tender in relieving his suffering patients, in as much as he himself must one day be a like sufferer."

—*Thomas Sydenham*

"A doctor must work eighteen hours a day and seven days a week. If you cannot console yourself to this, get out of the profession."

—*Martin H. Fischer*

"Financial ruin from medical bills is almost exclusively an American disease."

—*Roul Turley*

"The doctor who can no longer find time in his day for prayer and the inner life, time to prepare for his consultations in the presence of God and to seek his will for his patients, cannot bring to them the spiritual climate that is necessary if they are to open their hearts to him. Driven on by his devotion to the needs of his practice, he leads a fatiguing and unsatisfying life in which only more and more rarely does he find those peaceful moments on intimacy when he can provide what the patient most expects of him."

—*Paul Tournier*

"Compared with the small pond of knowledge in medicine, our ignorance is Atlantic."

—*William A. Silverman*

"Until a physician has killed one or two patients, he is not a good physician."

—*Kashmiri Proverb*

"The world does not need a new medicine; it needs doctors who know how to pray and obey God in their own lives. In such hands, medicine with all its modern resources, will bring forth fruits in abundance."

—Paul Tournier

"Educating the mind without educating the heart is no education at all."

—Aristotle

"Knowledge speaks but wisdom listens."

—Jimi Hendrix

"The best doctor is the one you run for and can't find."

—Diderot

"Do what you will, the time will probably come when you will want the advice of a physician. Choose a sensible man, personally agreeable to yourself, if possible whom you know to have had a good education, to stand well with the members of his own profession, and of whom other scientific men, as well as physicians, speak respectfully... Once having chosen your medical adviser, be slow to leave him, except for good cause. He has served as apprenticeship to your constitution."

—Oliver Wendell Holmes

"I am dying with the help of too many physicians."

—Alexander The Great

"...The medical student should possess a pleasant appearance and good looks with a well-proportioned body, which should be free from physical defects or any obvious diseases. Above all he must be compassionate. He must exhibit deep interest in the art and science of healing."

—Charaka Samhita

"... Someone other than our parents responsible for our birth, Someone we always turn to when we need real help,

Someone who advises, comforts, sympathizes and cares, Someone who loses his sleep to keep us hale and hearty, Someone we always forget the minute we're fine, Someone who seldom gets thanked for all he's done, Someone who practices the world's noblest profession."

–Ode to the Doctor

"Doctors don't know everything. They understand matter, not spirit. And you and I live in the spirit."

–William Saroyan

"The most essential part of a student's instruction is obtained not in the lecture-room, but at the bedside. Nothing seen there is lost, the rhythms of disease are learned by frequent repetition; its unforeseen occurrences stamp themselves indelibly in the memory."

–Oliver Wendell Holmes

"For the physician, it is undoubtedly an important recommendation to be of good appearance and well-fed, since people take the view that those who do not know how to look after their own bodies are in no position to look after those of others. He must know how and when to be silent and to live an ordered life, as this greatly enhances his reputation. His learning must be that of an honest man, for this he must be honest towards all people and kindly and understanding. He must not act impulsively or hastily; he must look calm, serene and never cross, on the other hand, it does not behove for him to be too jolly."

–Hippocrates

"Physicians and politicians resemble one another in this respect, that some defend the constitution and others destroy it."

–Anonymous

"A *vaidya* is an invincible warrior, because he fights the elements of death. A *vaidya* is the giver of life, and so he is cherished in nature."

—*Maharishi Mahesh Yogi*

"The practice of medicine will be very much as you make it—to one a worry, a care, a perpetual annoyance; to another, a daily job and a life of as much happiness and usefulness as can well fall to the lot of man, because it is a life of self-sacrifice and of countless opportunities to comfort and help the weak-hearted, and to raise up those that fall."

—*William Osler*

"Only that, which can bring about a cure is a power medicine, and only he who relieves his patients of their ailments is the foremost among physicians."

—*Charaka*

"If the license to practice meant the completion of his education, how sad it would be for the practitioner, how distressing to his patients! More clearly than any other, the physician should illustrate the truth of Plato's saying that education is a life-long process. The training of the medical school gives a man his direction, points him the way and furnishes a chart, fairly incomplete, for the voyage, but nothing more. Postgraduation study has always been a characteristic feature of our profession."

—*William Osler*

"We doctors have always been a simple, trusting folk! Did we not believe Galen implicity for fifteen hundred years and Hipprocrates for more than two thousand years?"

—*William Osler*

"No man is a good doctor who has never been sick himself."

—*Chinese Proverb*

"There are only two sorts of doctors; those who practice with their brains, and those who practice with their tongues."

−William Osler

"Let the young students know, they will never find a more interesting, more instructive book than the patient himself."

−Giorgio Baglivi

"When simple, earnest spirit animates a colleague, there is no appreciable interval between the teacher and the taught—both are in the same class, the one a little more advanced than the other."

−William Osler

"Modern medicine is a product of the Greek intellect, and had its origin when those wonderful people created positive or rational science."

−William Osler

"Physicians are rather like undescended testicles, they are difficult to locate and when they are found, they are pretty ineffective."

−Anonymous

"To me the ideal doctor would be a man endowed with profound knowledge of life and of the soul, intuitively divining any suffering or disorder of whatever kind, and restoring peace by his mere presence."

−Henri Amiel

"The daily round of a busy practitioner tends to develop an egoism of a most intense kind, to which there is no antidote. The mistakes are often buried, and successful work tends to make a man touchy, dogmatic, intolerant of correction and abominably self-centered. The medical society is the best corrective, and a man misses a good part of his education who does not get knocked about a bit by his colleagues in discussions and criticisms."

–William Osler

"The training of the medical school gives a man his direction, points him the way, and furnishes him with a chart, fairly incomplete, for the voyage, but nothing more."

–William Osler

"Perfect happiness for student and teacher will come with the abolition of examinations, which are stumbling blocks and rocks of offence in the pathway of the true student."

–William Osler

"It is astonishing with how after little reading a doctor can practise medicine, but it is not astonishing how badly he may do it."

–William Osler

"Students work to pass, not to know. They do pass and they don't know."

–Thomas Henry Huxley

"The practice of medicine is an art, not trade, a calling, not a business, a calling in which your heart will be exercised equally with your head."

–William Osler

"The art of the practice of medicine is to be learned only by experience; it's not an inheritance; it cannot be revealed."

–William Osler

"The student often resembles the poet—he is born, not made."

–William Osler

"The teacher's life should have three periods—study until 25, investigation until 40, profession until 60, at which age I would have him retired on a double allowance."

—*William Osler*

"The truth in medicine is an end that cannot be reached and all that is written in books is worth much less than the experience of a wise doctor."

—*Rhazes*

"To be a good doctor, sometimes you must envision yourself as slightly stupid, skeptical, curious and quizzical."

—*Gordon Mehler*

"Doctors are just the same as lawyers; the only difference is that lawyers merely rob you, whereas doctors rob you and kill you, too."

—*Anton Chekhov*

"Given one well-trained physician of the highest type and he will do better work for a thousand people than ten specialists."

—*William James Mayo*

"He is the best physician in whom the patient has the greatest confidence."

—*Peter Shaw*

"Doctors get money when they do procedures—family practice doesn't have any procedures...... We get nothing for use of our time to understand the lives of our patients. Technology is rewarded in medicine, it seems to one, and not thinking."

—*David Jones*

"A man is a poor physician who does not has two or three remedies ready for use in every case of illness."

—*Asclepiades*

"A physician is an unfortunate gentleman who is required everyday to perform a miracle; namely to reconcile health with intemperance."

—Voltaire

"Fifty years ago the successful doctor was said to need three attributes; a top hat to give him Authority, a paunch to give him Diginity, and piles to give him Axious expression."

—Anonymous

Prognosis

"Patients (and attendants) have emotional feelings. Never say, 'nothing can be done', because something can always be done. Never give a hopeless prognosis in order to avoid the neglect and to sustain the will to fight. Nevertheless be pragmatic."
–*Meharban Singh*

"The younger the patient, the worse the prognosis in diseases of childhood. This is in consequence of the feeble resistance of the infantile organism to all diseases particularly those, which are of an acute nature."
–*L. Emmett Holt*

"Those by nature overweight, die earlier than slim."
–*Hippocrates*

"Diseases with an acute and sudden onset are likely to have either a dramatic recovery or a deadly outcome."
–*Meharban Singh*

"A treatment method or an educational method that will work for one child, may not work for another child. The one common denominator for all the young children is that early intervention does work, and it seems to improve the prognosis."
–*Temple Grandin*

"We know from our clinical experience in the practice of medicine that in diagnosis, prognosis and treatment, the individual and his background of heredity are just as important, if not more so, as the disease itself."
–*Paul Dudley White*

Public Health

"Treating someone who is already ill is like beginning to dig a well after you have become thirsty."

—Chinese Proverb

"The aim of medicine is to prevent disease and prolong life; the ideal of medicine is to eliminate the need of a physician."

—William J. Mayo

"The aim of the art of medicine is health, but its end is the possession of health. Doctors have to know by which means to bring about health, when it is absent, and by which means to preserve it, when it is present."

—Galen

"Of all forms of inequality, injustice in health care is the most shocking and inhuman."

—Martin Luther King Jr

"Medicine is the science of which we learn the various states of the human body in health, when not in health, the means by which health is likely to be lost, and when lost, the means by which it is likely to be restored to health."

—Avicenna

"Immunization is one of the most cost-effective public health investments today."

—Lee Jong-Wook

"Society and government should work together to give priority to the poorest of the poor and make efforts to provide affordable health services."

–Narendra Modi

"An able physician is more useful to a patient than the most devoted friend, and progress in medical knowledge does more for the health of the community than ill-informed philanthropy."

–Bertrand Russell

"One of the first duties of the physician is to educate the masses not to take medicine."

–William Osler

"When meditating over a disease, I never think of finding a remedy for it. But instead I think of ways and means of preventing it."

–Louis Pasteur

"Prevention is better than cure."

–Erasmus

"He who cures a disease may be the skillfullest, but he that prevents it is the safest physician."

–Thomas Fuller

"An ounce of prevention is worth a pound of care."

–Bejamin Franklin

"Soap and water, and common sense are best disinfectants."

–William Osler

"Nine-tenths of our sickness can be prevented by right thinking plus right hygiene — nine-tenths of it!"

–Henry Miller

"Barn-yard medicine has not given us any vaccination procedure that really protects against illness, but many that endanger the body, that even bring death."

–Guttman

"The public is surely entitled to convincing proof, beyond all reasonable doubt, that artificial immunization is in fact a safe and effective procedure, in no way injurious to health, and that the threat of the corresponding natural diseases remain sufficiently clear and urgent to warrant mass inoculation of everyone, even against their will if necessary. Unfortunately, such proof has never been given."

–Richard Moskowitz

"Let everyone sweep infront of his own door; and the whole world will be clean."

–Goethe

"How far can a mother walk with a sick baby in her arms? Health care must be available within that distance."

–Abhay Bang

"The public blabbers about preventive medicine, but will neither appreciate nor pay for it. You get paid for what you cure."

–Martin H. Fischer

"I hope some day the practice of producing cowpox in humans will spread over the world—when that day comes, there will be no more smallpox."

–Edward Jenner

"Meat consumption is just as dangerous to public health as tobacco use…… It's time we looked into holding the meat producers, and fast-food outlets legally accountable."

–Neal Barnard

"Cleanliness is indeed next to godliness."
–John Wesley

"It does not require money to be neat, clean and dignified."
–Mahatma Gandhi

"Doctors are health care providers, not health cure providers."
–Anonymous

"If each one of us would only sweep infront of own door step, the whole world would be cleaner."
–Mother Teresa

"And I believe that the best buy in public health today must be a combination of regular physical exercise and a healthy diet."
–Julie Bishop

"In this country doctors are, as a rule, bad citizens, taking little or no interest in civic, state or national politics. Let me tell of one of us who found time to serve his city and his country. For more than twenty years Virchow sat in the Berlin City Council as an alderman, and to no feature in his extraordinary life does the Berliner point with more justifiable pride. It is a combination of qualities only too rare, when the learned professor can leave his laboratory and take his share in practical, municipal work."
–William Osler

"We don't know what is going to happen but we do know if there is a pandemic, people need to be prepared. Preparedness starts now."
–Rami Yoakum

"We need to start training more primary health care providers and fewer specialists. We will never be able to control health care costs unless we challenge the over-emphasis on medical research, specialist and technology, and put more emphasis on delivering good, everyday basic medicine to those who now have none."

–Richard Lamm

"Mainstream medicine would be way different if they focused on prevention even half as much as they focused on intervention."

–Anonymous

"Listen to children and ensure their participation. Children and adolescents are resourceful citizens capable of helping to build a better future for all. We must respect their right to express themselves and to participate in all matters affecting them, in accordance with their age and maturity."

–Declaration of A World Fit for Children 2002

"Coitus interruptus: copulation without population."

–Anonymous

"The enhancement of neonatal and infant survival is truly the key to the success of family welfare program and stabilization of population dynamics which is a major public health issue in India."

–Meharban Singh

"Physical activity is one of the most undervalued interventions to improve public health. Physical activity is closely associated with better health and reduced all cause mortality, including reduced mortality from coronary heart disease, stroke, colon cancer and reduced fatality after a heart attack."

–Liam Donaldson

"Depression has been called the world's number one public health problem. In fact depression is so widespread, it is considered as the common cold of psychiatric disturbances. But there is a grim difference between depression and a cold. Depression can kill you."

–David D. Burns

"Smokers smoke because they are addicted to nicotine in cigarettes, but it is the smoke, not the nicotine, which causes long list of diseases, including lung cancer, heart disease, stroke and emphysema."

–Richard Daines

"In a democracy the ultimate responsibility for decisions on health policy should be with the public."

–Geoffery Rose

"Every year 13 to 20 billion dollars could he saved in health care costs by demedicalising childbirth, developing midwifery, and encouraging breastfeeding."

–Frank A. Oski

"Advances in medicine and agriculture have saved vastly more lives than have been lost in all the wars in history."

–Carl Sagan

Research, Publications and Teaching

24

"A bit of science distances one from God, but much of science nears one to Him...... The more I study nature, the more I stand amazed at the work of the Creator."

—Louis Pasteur

"When you publish something, it is very much as if you have pulled your pants down in public. If what you have written is good, nobody can hurt you; if what you have written is bad, no body can help you."

—Edna St. Vincent Millay

"Educating the mind without educating the heart is no education at all."

—Aristotle

"The author who speaks about his own books is almost as bad as a mother who talks about her own children."

—Benjamin Disraeli

"The twenty thousand biomedical journals now published are increasing by six to seven percent a year. To review ten journals in internal medicine, a physician must read about two hundred articles and seventy editorials a month."

—Phil Manning

"A home without books is a body without soul."

—Cicero

"Brevity in writing is the best insurance for its perusal."
—*Rudolph Virchow*

"Teach the tongue to say, 'I do not know'."
—*Talmud*

"I have been trying to point out that in our lines, chance may have an astonishing influence, and if I may offer advice to the young laboratory worker, it would be this—never to neglect an extraordindary appearance or happening."
—*Alexander Fleming*

"The light microscope opened the first gate to microcosm. The electron microscope opened the second gate to microcosm. What will one find opening the third gate?"
—*Ernst Ruska*

"Stem cell research can revolutionize medicine, more than anything since discovery of antibiotics."
—*Ron Reagan*

"Science is father of knowledge, but opinion breeds ignorance."
—*Hippocrates*

"Some books are to be tasted, others to be swallowed and few to be chewed and digested."
—*Francis Bacon*

"A drug is that substance which, when injected into a rat, will produce a scientific report."
—*Author Unknown*

"Teaching and research are the warp and woof of the fabric of medical progress. Each is dependent on the other. The importance of both is now well recognised by medical schools and research institutes alike."
—*James B. Herrick*

"Research is subordinated (not to a long-term social benefit) but to an immediate commercial profit. Currently, disease (not health) is one of the major sources of profit for the pharmaceutical industry, and the doctors are willing agents of those profits."

—Pierre Bosquet

"The evolution of knowledge is towards simplicity and not complexity."

—L. Ron Hubbard

"Brevity is the best recommendation of a speech, whether by a senator or an orator."

—Cicero

"Medical education does not exist to provide students with a way of making a living, but to ensure the health of the community."

—Rudolph Virchow

"Those who have dissected or inspected many bodies have at least learnt to doubt, while others who are ignorant of anatomy and do not take trouble to attend to it, are in no doubt at all."

—Giovanni Bathista Morgagni

"The work of the doctor will, in the future, be ever more that of an educator, and ever less than that of a man who treats ailments."

—Lord Horder

"A peculiar thing in medicine is that we never believe in anything unless it can be demonstrated in animals."

—John A. Schindler

"If you steal from one author, it is plagiarism. If you steal from many, it's research."

—Wilson Miznor

"Half of what is true today will be proven to be incorrect in the next five years. Unfortunately, we don't know which half that is going to be."

–G. Lakshipati

"Five years after you finish medical school, everything you were taught will be wrong; but if you wait an additional five years it will be right again."

–Anonymous

"Don't think of organ donations as giving up part of yourself to keep a total stranger alive. It's really a total stranger giving up almost all of himself to keep part of you alive."

–Author Unknown

"Any intelligent fool can make things bigger and more complex. It takes a touch of genius and lot of courage to move to the opposite direction."

–Albert Einstein

"I hear and I forget. I see and I remember. I do and I understand."

–Confucius

"He who asks may be a fool for five minutes. He who doesn't is a fool for lifetime."

–Chinese Saying

"All we know is still infinitely less than all that remains unknown."

–William Harvey

"I don't believe medical discoveries are doing much to advance human life. As fast as we create ways to extend it, we are inventing ways to shorten it.

–Christiaan Barnard

"Too much attention to health is a hindrance to learning to invention and to studies of any kind. Because we are always feeling suspicious and blame our studies for everything."

–Plato

"There are three kinds of lies: lies, damned lies and statistics."

–Benjamin Disraeli

"...Medical research is subject to ethical standards that promotes respect for all human beings and protect their health and rights. Research investigators should be aware of the ethical, legal and regulatory requirements for research on human subjects in their own countries as well as applicable to international requirements. Medical research is only justified if there is a reasonable likelihood that the populations in which the research is carried out stand to benefit from the results of the research...."

–World Medical Association
Declaration of Helsinki, 2000

"It is science alone that can solve the problems of hunger and poverty, insanitation and illiteracy, harmful superstitions, customs and traditions. The vast resources are being wasted in a rich country inhabited by starving people—the future belongs to science."

–Jawaharlal Nehru

"Statistics don't lie, liars use statistics."

–Mark Twain

"Dolly's death confirms what we all know, which is that there are problems with cloning. Cloning is still just as much an art as a science."

–Robert Lanza

"Medical statistics are like a bikini bathing suit; what they reveal is interesting, what they conceal is vital."

–Anonymous

"The most important of my discoveries have been suggested to me by my failures."

–*Humphry Davy*

"It is my ambition to say in ten sentences what others say in a whole book."

–*Friedrich Nietzsche*

"All truths are easy to understand once they are discovered; the point is to discover them."

–*Galileo Galilei*

"Examinations are formidable even to the best prepared, for the greatest fool may ask more than the wisest man can offer."

–*Charles C. Colton*

"The science of life shall never attain finality. Therefore, humility and relentless industry should characterize your every endeavor and approach to knowledge. The entire world consist of teachers for the wise and enemies for the fools. Therefore, knowledge, conducive to health, longevity, fame and excellence coming even from an unfamiliar source should be received, assimilated and utilized with earnestness."

–*Charak Samhita*

"Get accustomed to test all sorts of book problems and statements for yourself, and take as little as possible on trust. The Hunterian 'Do not think, but try' attitude of mind is the important one to cultivate."

–*William Osler*

"Should your assistant make an important observation, let him publish it. Through your students and your disciples will come your greatest honor."

–*William Osler*

"Information is not knowledge, knowledge is not wisdom and wisdom is not foresight. Each grows out of the other and we need them all."

—Arthur Clarke

"The secret of a good lecture is to have a good beginning and a good ending, and to have the two as close together as possible."

—George Burns

"When you do the common things in life in an uncommon way, you will command the attention of the world."

—George Washington Carver

"The safest thing for a patient is to be in the hand of a man engaged in teaching medicine. In order to be a teacher of medicine, the doctor must always be a student."

—Charles Mayo

"We cannot teach people anything, we can only help them discover it within themselves."

—Galileo Galilei

"I am not accustomed to saying anything with certainty after only one or two observations."

—Andreas Vesalius

"In the real world, 90% of the money spent on medical research is focused on conditions that are responsible for just 10% of the deaths and disability caused by diseases globally."

—Peter Singer

"I desire no other epitaph than the statement that I taught medical students in the wards, as I regard this as by far the most useful and important work I have been called upon to do."

—William Osler

"An understanding heart is everything in a teacher and cannot be esteemed highly enough. One looks back with appreciation to the brilliant teachers but with gratitude to those who touched our human feeling."

–Carl Jung Gustav

25

Specialists and Experts

"A specialist is a man who knows more and more about less and less until he knows everything about nothing. A general practitioner is one who knows less and less about more and more until he knows nothing about everything. It is true that more we learn, the less we understand and eventually a stage will come when we will know everything but understand nothing."

–Anonymous

"What Nissl and Alzheimer could find under their microscopes they declared "neurology." What they couldn't find was psychiatry."

–Edward Shorter

"*Psychiatry*: The care of the id by the odd."

–Anon

"The human body is the only machine for which there are no spare parts."

–Hermann M. Biggs

"A surgeon should be young, a physician old."

–French Proverb

"Anyone who goes to a psychiatrist should have his head examined."

–Samuel Goldwyn

"Some tortures are physical, and some are mental. But the one that is both is dental."

—Ogden Nash

"Experimental psychologist: A scientist who pulls habits out of rats."

—Leonard Louis Levinson

"The consultant is one, who sees the patient at a time when he is already on the road to recovery."

—Meharban Singh

"You go to a psychiatrist when you're slightly cracked and keep going until you're completely broke."

—Anonymous

"Expert is one who knows more and more about less and less."

—Nicholas Murray Butler

"A psychologist once said that we know little about the conscience except that it is soluble in alcohol."

—Thomas Blackburn

"Physicians of the utmost fame were called urgently. But when they came they answered as they took their fees—there is no cure for this disease."

—Hilaire Belloc

"It's better than riches, to scratch when it itches."

—Author Unknown

"What do you call two orthopedic surgeons reading an EKG? A double blind study."

—Anonymous

"Neurosis is always a substitute for legitimate suffering."

—Carl Jung Gustav

"You cannot afford to stand aloof from your professional colleagues in any place. Join their associations, mingle in their meetings, giving of the best of your talents, gathering here, scattering there; but everywhere showing that you are at all times faithful student, as willing to teach as to be taught."

—William Osler

"Happiness is your dentist telling you it won't hurt and then having him catch his hand in the drill."

—Johny Carson

"A psychiatrist is a man who goes to a striptease club and watches the audience."

—Merve Stockwood

"The only differences between psychiatrists and their patients is that the patients have a chance of getting better."

—Anonymous

"Fingerprints cannot lie, but liars can make fingerprints."

—Popular Saying

"The corpse is a silent witness who never lies."

—Anonymous

"A person's fingerprint is like a biological seal, once impressed, can never be denied."

—Colin Beavan

"Homeopathy is based on the Hippocrates law of similar, i.e. like cures like. By giving the body a substance (in an infinitesimal dose) that produces the same effect as the disease, it would ultimately enable the body to overcome the disease."

—Samuel Hahnemann

"Show me a sane man and I will cure him for you."
—*Carl Jung Gustav*

"The science of psychiatry is now where the science of medicine was before germs were discovered."
—*Malcolm Rogers*

"Where I'd was, there ego shall be."
—*Sigmund Freud*

"A physician is someone who knows everything and does nothing."

A surgeon is someone who does everything and knows nothing.

A psychiatrist is someone who knows nothing and does nothing.

A pathologist is someone who knows everything and does everything too late."
—*Anonymous*

"One of my surgical friends had in his operation room a sign. 'If the operation is difficult, you aren't doing it right.' What he meant was, you have to plan every operation. You cannot ever be casual and you have to realize that any operation is a potential fatality."
—*Joseph E. Murray*

"There are in truth, no specialties in medicine, since to know fully many of the most important diseases, a physician must be familiar with their manifestations in many organs."
—*William Osler*

"We must admit that we have never fought the homeopathy on matters of principle. We fought them becuase they came into our community and got the business."
—*JN McCormack*

"It is illogical to treat a patient simultaneously with a homeopathic as well as an allopathic medicine because one is supposed to express the disease and the other tries to suppress it."

–Meharban Singh

"I find most men would rather have their bellies opened for five hundred dollars than have a tooth pulled out for five ."

–Martin H. Fischer

"I was never afraid of anything in the world except the dentist."

–Taylor Caldwell

"A certain degree of neurosis is of inestimable value as a drive, especially to a psychologist."

–Sigmund Freud

"My idea is that it is better even to die under the treatment of a scientific doctor than expect recovery from the treatment by laymen who know nothing of modern science but blindly go by the ancient books."

–Swami Vivekananda

26

Surgeons and Surgical Procedures

"I think circumcision is a good idea... . However, it is not absolutely necessary. I strongly recommend leaving the foreskin alone."

—Benjamin Spock

"If non-therapeutic child circumcision were a new drug, the FDA would never approve it. If it were proposed a new surgical procedure, it would never be approved."

—David Gollaher

"If I was to cut off any other part of a baby for no good cause and without an anesthetic, I'd be struck off the medical register and the parents would most likely lose custody of the child."

—Christopher Green

"Until the child is old enough to participate in the decision, we should not do any cosmetic surgery."

—Bruce E. Wilson

"If I was a newborn baby tonight and I could speak and I was asked about circumcision, I would say, 'Can you hold off a bit until I can make up my own mind'."

—Roger McClay

"The most wonderful thing you can do is to give the gift of sight. Talk with your family about becoming an organ donor."

—Benjamin Harris

"Of all the things that it is possible to donate, to donate your own body is infinetely more worthwhile."

—Manusmriti

"She got her good looks from her father. He's a plastic surgeon."

—Groucho Marx

"They had me on the operating table all day. They looked into my stomach, my gall bladder, they examined everything inside of me. Know what they decided? I need glasses."

—Joe E. Lewis

"Don't take your organs to heaven with you. Heaven knows we need them here."

—Author Unknown

"A very bold surgeon is the one who realizes that his patient takes all the risks."

—Anonymous

"Surgery, like making love must be done gently with adequate exposure."

—Anonymous

"It takes five years to learn when to operate and twenty years to learn when not to."

—Anonymous

"The practice of medicine is a thinker's art, the practice of surgery, a plumber's."

—Martin H. Fischer

"Before undergoing a surgical operation, arrange your temporal affairs. You may live."

—Ambrose Bierce

"When in doubt, blame anesthesia (or an anesthesiologist!)"

—Anonymous

"The lesser the indication for surgery, the greater the complications."

–Anonymous

"A patient is never too sick for a life saving procedure."

–Anonymous

"A hospital should also have a recovery room adjoining the cashier's office."

–Francis O. Walsh

"Measure thrice, think twice, cut once."

–Anonymous

"Surgeon can cut everything except cause."

–Herbert M. Shelton

"Surgery is 70% scut work, 20% boredom, and 10% learning."

–Anonymous

"I got the bill for my surgery. Now I know what those doctors were wearing masks for."

–James H. Boren

"Surgery is learned with the hands and the eyes and not by studying books while sitting comfortably in your chair."

–Ambroise Pare

"A good surgeon must have an eagle's eye, a lion's heart and a lady's hand."

–Anonymous

"The frequency of disastrous consequences in compound fracture, contrasted with the complete immunity from danger to life or limb in simple fracture, is one of the most striking as well as melancholy facts in surgical practice."

–Joseph Lister

"I learnt a long time ago that minor surgery is when they do the operation on someone else, not you."

–Bill Walton

"I don't dawdle I'm a surgeon. I make an incision, do what needs to be done and sew up the wound. There is a beginning, a middle and an end."

–Richard Selzer

"A surgeon should give as little pain as possible while he is treating the patient and no pain at all when he charges his fee."

–Anonymous

"As a surgeon you have to have a controlled arrogance. If it's uncontrolled, you kill people, but you have to be pretty arrogant to saw through a person's chest, take out their heart and believe you can fix it. Then, when you succeed and the patient survives, you pray, because it's only the grace of God that you get there."

–Mehmet Oz

"Every surgeon carries within himself a small cemetery, where from time to time he goes to pray—a place of bitterness and regret, where he must look for an explanation for his failures."

–Rene Leriche

Source Materials

1. Adams F. The Genuine Works of Hippocrates. Baltimore, The Williams and Wilkins Co, 1939.

2. Apley John, MacKeith Ronald, Meadow Roy. The Child and his Symptoms. London, Blackwell Scientific Publications, 3rd edition, 1978.

3. Apley John. Pediatrics. London, Bailliere Tindall, 2nd edition, 1979.

4. Bartlett J. Familiar Quotations. Boston, Little Brown Co, 17th edition, 1968.

5. Bean RB, Bean WB (Eds.). Sir William Osler: Aphorisms from His Bedside Teachings and Writings. Springfield, IL; Charles C Thomas, 1961.

6. Bryson Alan. Healing Mind, Body and Soul. New Delhi; Sterling Publications, 1999.

7. Carper Jean. Food: Your Miracle Medicine. New York; Harper Perennial, 1994.

8. Carper Jean. Your Miracle Brain. New York; Harper Collins Publishers, 2000.

9. Chadwick J, Mann WN. The Medical Works of Hippocrates. Oxford, Blackwell Scientific Publications, 1950.

10. Chopra Deepak. Quantum Healing. New York, Bantam Books, 1990.

11. Cushing Harvey. The Life of Sir William Osler, 2 volumes. Oxford; The Clarendon Press, 1925.

12. Gordon Richard. Quantum Touch: The Power to Heal. New Delhi, New Age Books, 2001.

13. Harvey A McGehee, McKusick Victor A. Osler's Textbook Revisited. New York, Appleton-Century-Crofts, 1967.

14. John Alfred. Dictionary of Quotations. New Delhi, New Light Publishers, 2001.

15. Johnson Rex, Swindley David. Awaken your Inner Power. Boston, Element Books Ltd, 1995.

16. Lewis Paul. History of Medicine. Chancellor Press, 2001.

17. Malhotra Meera. Orient Book of Quotations. New Delhi, Orient Paper Backs, 1976.

18. Moyers Bill. Healing and the Mind. New York; Main Street Books, 1993.

19. Osho. Joy: the Happiness that Comes from Within. New York, St. Martin's Griffins, 2004.

20. Robbins Anthony. Awaken the Giant Within. New York, Simon and Schuster, 1991.

21. Roland Charles G. Sir William Osler 1849–1919: A selection for medical students. Toronto, The Hannah Institute for the History of Medicine, 1982.

22. Roy Stemman. Healers and Healing. London, Judy Piatkus Ltd., 1999.

23. Sharma Robin S. Mega Living. Mumbai, Jaico Publishing House, 2003.

24. Siegel Bernie. Peace, Love and Healing. London, Rider, 1982.

25. Siegal Bernie. Love, Medicine and Miracles. London, Random House, 1986.

26. Singh Meharban. Pediatric Clinical Methods. New Delhi, CBS Publishers & Distributors Pvt Ltd, 5th edition, 2016.

27. Singh Meharban. Care of the Newborn. New Delhi, CBS Publishers & Distributors Pvt Ltd, 8th edition, 2015.

28. Singh Meharban. The Pearls of Wisdom and Art of Living. New Delhi, Sagar Publications, 1st edition, 2007.

29. The New International Webster's Comprehensive Dictionary. Trident Press International 1996, p1845–1895.

30. Thondup Tulku. The Healing Power of Mind. Boston, Shambhala, 1996.

31. Tolle Eckhart. The Power of Now. Mumbai, Yogi Impressions Books Pvt. Ltd., 2001.

Index